The New Bodybuilder Cookbook 2021

Beginners Edition

CONTENTS

CHAPTER 1: MUSCLE IS WON OR LOST IN THE KITCHEN

Many experts feel that your nutritional habits make for up to 80% of the way your body looks. Every drip of sweat and effort you exude in the gym is wasted if your nutrition is not on point. If you want to build a substantial amount of muscle and strength or lose fat then you must fuel your body accordingly.

EATING FOR MUSCLE

To build muscle, you need to take in an excess of calories with the right nutrients to grow. If you don't eat enough, your body won't be able to fully repair the damage you cause by lifting weights, triggering you to plateau or even worse, lose muscle. However don't make the mistake most gym rats make by eating everything in sight, from pizzas to pop-tarts, as this is extremely unhealthy in the long-term. As you'll see from the upcoming recipes, eating the right foods doesn't have to be boring, bland or time–consuming.

EATING TO SHRED

To lose fat, you need to take in fewer calories than you expend. Again if you don't take in the right nutrients and foods, you will lose muscle. Losing fat generally requires you to be more precise which leads to many adopting the "Chicken, Rice and Broccoli diet," which is incredible boring, bland and usually leads to many people failing.

I created these recipes to escape the tedious, boring diets that many gym-goers subject themselves to and to finally make dieting enjoyable.

CHAPTER 2: THE FUNDAMENTAL PILLARS OF A MUSCLE BUILDING/FAT BURNING DIET

Before you ask, you won't need to be a qualified nutritionist to create your perfect diet. You just need to understand a few simple things:

1. What Protein, Carbohydrates and Fats are and what they're used for.

2. How much you need of each and what foods you'll get them from.

3. How many calories you need to achieve your goals of either building muscle or burning fat.

WHAT IS PROTEIN?

Protein is used by your body for a number of processes from enzyme and hormone production to ensuring your immune system is working optimally. The reason why protein is so important in a muscle building diet is because protein is absolutely critical for muscle growth and repair. Working out and 'tearing down muscle' increases your body's demand for protein. As you build more and more muscle, the more protein your body will require to repair, grow and maintain that muscle. If you don't supply your body with enough protein, it will take it from your muscles causing muscle breakdown. Making sure you get enough protein is therefore of upmost importance in planning your diet.

WHAT ARE CARBOHYDRATES?

Carbohydrates get converted into glucose and then are used by your body for energy. There are two types of carbohydrates - simple and complex. Simple carbohydrates are foods like fruit, white rice and sugar. Complex carbohydrates are foods like sweet potatoes, brown rice and vegetables. Complex carbohydrates tend to be thought of as the better of the two. The difference between these types of carbohydrates is how long it takes the body to convert them into glucose. Simple carbohydrates are converted by your body quickly making them great for a fast source of energy however there is usually a fast decline after. It takes your body a lot longer to convert complex carbohydrates into glucose making them a much more sustaining source of energy. The reason so many people are afraid of carbohydrates is because whatever your body doesn't use gets moved into your fat stores. Carbohydrates however are not the enemy and are vital for your success.

WHAT ARE FATS?

Fats are vital for many of your bodily functions. They are needed for the production of many hormones in your body and they also help keep your brain and nervous system running optimally. They are also the most calorically dense out of the three macronutrients – every gram of fat contains 9 calories!

There are four types of fat: Monounsaturated, Polyunsaturated, Saturated and

Trans-fatty acids. The only one you need to avoid is Trans-Fatty acids. These are fats that have been modified in a lab to ensure a longer shelf life. The body does not know what to do with them and therefore they can get into your cells and cause damage. They're most commonly found in packaged meals and used in many fried foods.

How much do you need of each?

Well that depends on your goals!

TO BUILD MUSCLE, A GOOD PLACE TO START FROM IS:

Protein = 1.5 grams per pound of bodyweight

Carbohydrates = 2 grams per pound of bodyweight

Fats = 0.5 grams per pound of bodyweight

You want to be gaining about 0.5 – 1 pound a week. Any more than that and you will be gaining too much fat. If you find you aren't gaining weight, increase your calories by around 100-200 calories each week until you reach the sweet spot. Alternatively if you're gaining too much, then you want to reduce your calories by around 100 – 200 each week.

TO MAINTAIN MUSCLE, A GOOD PLACE TO START FROM IS:

Protein= 1 gram per pound of bodyweight

Carbohydrates = 1 gram per pound of bodyweight

Fats = 0.5 grams per pound of bodyweight

TO LOSE WEIGHT, A GOOD PLACE TO START FROM IS:

Protein = 2 grams per pound of bodyweight

Carbohydrates = 0.5 grams per pound of bodyweight

Fats = 1 gram per pound of bodyweight

You want to be losing about 1 – 2 pound a week. Any more than that and you risk losing that hard earned muscle. If you find you aren't losing weight, decrease your calories by around 100-200 calories each week until you reach the sweet spot. Alternatively if you're losing too much, then you want to increase your calories by around 100 – 200 each week.

CHAPTER 3: THE TOP COMMANDMENTS OF GOOD NUTRITION

What you put into your body will either make or break the results you get in the gym. These are rules you must live by if you want to be successful in your muscle building and fat loss pursuits.

1. HAVE PROTEIN WITH EVERY MEAL

Protein is vital to your success if building or maintaining muscle mass is your goal. Aim to have a least 1 source of quality protein with every meal. At a minimum, you must aim for at least 1 pound of protein per pound of bodyweight.

2. THERE MUST BE GREEN ON THE PLATE

Vegetables contain so many essential nutrients that you simply can't get anywhere else. Aim to have at least 1 serving of vegetables with every meal.

3. FAT IS NOT EVIL

Let's get one thing straight; fat will not make you fat. If you want to build muscle and burn fat, it's vital that you get enough. As we've established, healthy fats are needed for the production of many hormones in your body including testosterone. The only fats you need to avoid are trans fats.

4. DON'T RELY ON SUPPLEMENTS, EAT 'REAL' FOOD

Supplements are meant to supplement your diet not make up the bulk of it. Aim to have at least 70% of your diet come from 'real' food.

5. STICK TO SLOW DIGESTING CARBS MOST OF THE TIME (EXCEPT AROUND YOUR WORKOUTS)

Slow digesting carbohydrates ensure a steady supply of energy and have less of an impact on your blood sugar levels. Regular consumption of fast digesting carbs has been linked to an increased risk of diabetes, heart disease and obesity. However after training, you want to replace your depleted glycogen stores quickly as this can prevent your body becoming catabolic and keep you in a "muscle building" state. This is why you would want to consume a fast digesting carbohydrate after your workout.

6. DRINK WATER AND LOTS OF IT

It is absolutely essential to drink enough water. When you don't get enough, performance can be severely affected. Therefore try to get in about 3 – 4 litres of pure, clean water per day.

Okay so now you know the science, let's get cooking!

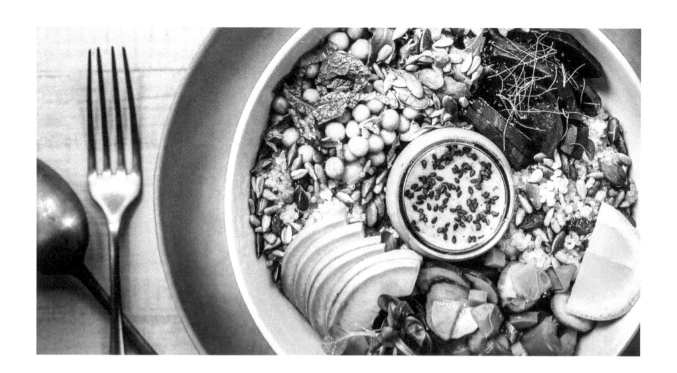

BREAKFAST

It's the most important meal of the day. Your parents told you. Your teachers told you. And now you know it. How can you expect not to have a total burn out, or beat your PB, or even have the energy to get your ass off the sofa if you haven't fuelled the machine? You can't. So use these quick, easy and tasty recipes to get you going. And no, it's not all raw eggs...

CHAPTER 4: BREAKFAST

MASS BUILDING SWEET POTATO PANCAKES

Start your day with this quick and easy, delicious protein packed pancake recipe. It contains all the right ingredients to keep you going and more than enough protein for your muscles to feast on!

Nutritional value

Calories per serving: 451,
Protein: 38g
Carbs: 74g
Fat: 9g

Ingredients

- 1 medium sized sweet potato
- 1 egg
- 4 egg whites
- 100g fat-free Greek yogurt
- 40g of oats
- 1 tsp cinnamon
- 1 tsp vanilla extract
- 1 tsp of honey
- Handful of diced strawberries
- Handful of blueberries

How to make:

1. Rinse sweet potato under cold water for a couple of seconds and then pierce it with a fork several times and place it in the microwave until soft (about 8 minutes).
2. After let it cool down before removing all skin with a knife.
3. Put the oats into a blender and blend until they are a fine powder, then place into a bowl.
4. Place the sweet potato in the blender and blend until smooth, and then mix with the powdered oats.
5. Add the egg, egg whites, vanilla, cinnamon, honey and yogurt and

stir well. This is now your pancake batter.

6. Spray a pan with cooking spray and place over medium heat. Pour roughly a quarter of the batter into the pan and cook for 1-2 minutes.

7. Flip the pancake and cook for another 30 seconds. Once done, remove your tasty pancake and top with the berries. Use the same method for the rest of your batter.

BRAWNY BREAKFAST BURRITO

Add a bit spice to your life with this Mexican inspired burrito. Contains great sources of protein, healthy fats and fibre to ensure you're building muscle the lean way.

Nutritional value

Calories per serving: 302
Protein: 25g
Carbs: 19g
Fat: 16g

Ingredients

• 2 eggs
• 50ml of low fat milk
• 25g of black beans
• 50g of low fat cheese
• Handful of chopped red peppers
• 1 tsp of chopped coriander
• 1 tbsp of salsa
• ½ tsp of cumin

How to make:

1. Add the milk, eggs and cumin to a bowl and whisk together.
2. Spray pan with cooking spray and place over medium heat. Add the mixture to the pan.
3. After roughly 2 – 3 minutes, add the low fat cheese, chopped red peppers and black beans to the omelette.
4. Once added fold the omelette in half and let it cook through (1-2 minutes).
5. Remove from pan and serve with the salsa and coriander.

SUPER SCRAMBLED TURKEY BACON EGGS ON TOAST

Mix up your boring egg based breakfasts with this delicious recipe. Eggs are a great source of complete protein as they contain all eight amino acids.

Nutritional value

(Serves 2)
Calories per serving: 299
Protein: 22g
Carbs: 35g
Fat: 8g

Ingredients

- 6 egg whites
- 3 slices of turkey bacon
- 2 slices of Ezekiel or wholemeal bread
- Handful of chopped onion
- Handful of chopped yellow peppers
- Handful of chopped white mushrooms
- 1 tsp of garlic powder
- 1 tsp of dried parsley
- 1 tsp of olive oil

How to make:

1. Spray pan with cooking spray and place over medium/high heat. Add the chopped onions, chopped yellow peppers and white mushrooms and cook until soft.
2. In a different pan, cook the turkey bacon.
3. Add the egg whites and garlic powder to the pan with the veggies and 1tsp of olive oil and scramble until the eggs become firm.
4. Toast the Ezekiel bread.
5. Break up the turkey bacon and add to the scrambled eggs
6. Plate up and serve scrambled eggs and turkey bacon on bread, sprinkled with the fresh parsley.

7. Add salt and pepper as required.

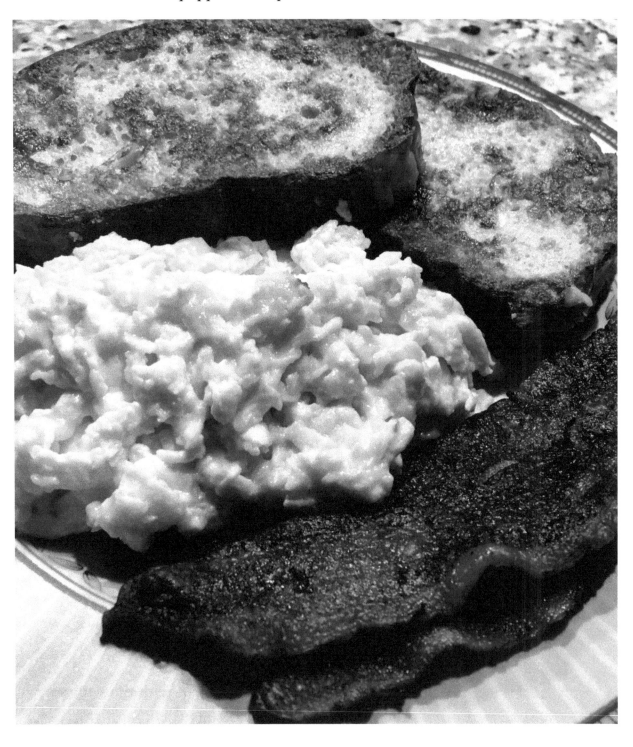

BANANA AND ALMOND MUSCLE OATMEAL

If you're in a hurry, this recipe is great. It takes around 5 minutes to make and still has the right macronutrients to make this a healthy and sustaining meal.

Nutritional value

Calories per serving: 523
Protein: 32g
Carbs: 60g
Fat: 15g

Ingredients

- 50g of rolled oats
- 200ml of low fat milk
- 1 scoop of whey protein (vanilla or chocolate)
- Handful of chopped almonds
- 1 tsp of organic peanut butter
- 1 diced banana

How to make:

1. Throw the oats and low fat milk into a large bowl, stir and place in the microwave for two minutes.
2. Add the diced banana, peanut butter, whey protein and chopped almonds to the oats and mix in.

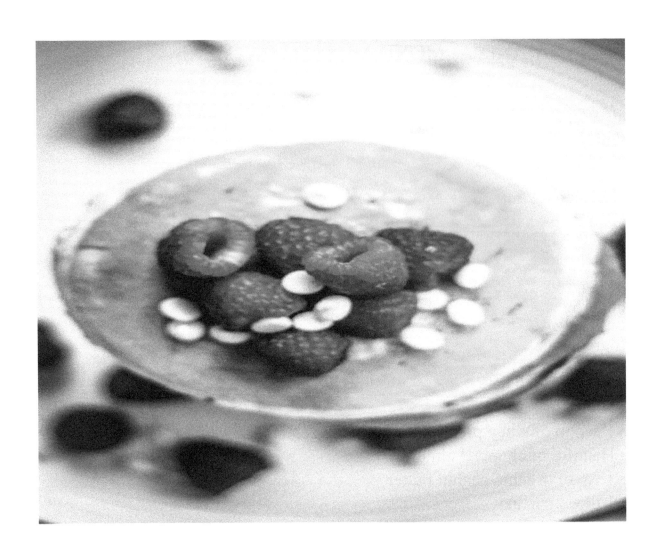

PROTEIN POWERED PANCAKES

If you're not a fan of sweet potato, then these are a great alternative. Lots of protein and quick and easy to make.

Nutritional value

(Makes about 5 pancakes)
Calories per serving: 337
Protein: 27g
Carbs: 33g
Fat: 9g

Ingredients

- 6 egg whites
- 40g of rolled oats
- 1 tsp flaxseed oil
- 1 tsp of cinnamon
- 1 tsp of stevia

  - Handful of small fruit of your choice to serve with

How to make:

1. Put the oats and all the other ingredients into a blender and blend. This is now your pancake batter.
2. Spray pan with cooking spray and place over medium heat.
3. Pour roughly 1/5 of the pancake batter into the pan and cook for 1-2 minutes. Flip the pancake and cook for another 30 seconds.
4. Once done, remove your tasty pancake.
5. Use the same method for the rest of your batter.
6. Serve with fruit of your choice

TURKEY MUSCLE OMELETTE

If you're looking for a protein packed, low carb meal for breakfast then this is it. Contains 26 grams of protein and only 5 grams of carbs.

Nutritional value

(Serves 2)
Calories per serving: 358
Protein: 26g
Carbs: 5g
Fat: 21g

Ingredients

- 150g of chopped or minced turkey
- 3 eggs
- Handful of baby spinach
- Handful of kale
- 1 tbsp of olive oil
- 25g of low fat cheese

How to make:

1. Crack the eggs into a bowl and whisk.
2. Grab a pan and heat half the oil on a medium heat, then add the turkey, kale and cheese and cook for 5-6 minutes.
3. In a different pan, heat the rest of the olive oil and then add the eggs and cook for around 4 minutes.
4. Add the turkey mix into the pan with the eggs and sprinkle some baby spinach on top, then fold the omelette in half.
5. Cook for another 2-3 minutes.
6. Plate up and serve.

AESTHETIC ASPARAGUS FRITTATA

A high protein and low carb breakfast which is great for those who are looking to minimize their carb intake.

Nutritional value

(Serves 3)
Calories per serving: 349
Protein: 23g
Carbs: 8g
Fat: 25g

Ingredients

- 300g of chopped asparagus
- ½ broccoli (florets only)
- 8 eggs
- Handful of chopped parsley
- 1 tsp of chives
- 1 tbsp of olive oil
- 100ml of low fat milk
- Salt and pepper

How to make:

1. Crack the eggs into a bowl, add the milk and some salt and pepper and whisk.
2. Get a covered skillet and steam the broccoli over a medium heat for 4-5 minutes. Set to one side.
3. Next, in the same skillet, heat the oil. Add the chopped asparagus, chopped parsley and chives into the skillet and cook for around 2-3 minutes on a medium heat.
4. Add the egg mixture, along with the broccoli into the skillet and cover the skillet evenly.
5. Cook for around 3-4 minutes or until the eggs are set right through
6. Take the skillet and place under the grill for around 2 minutes or

until the top is golden (optional).
7. Plate up and serve.

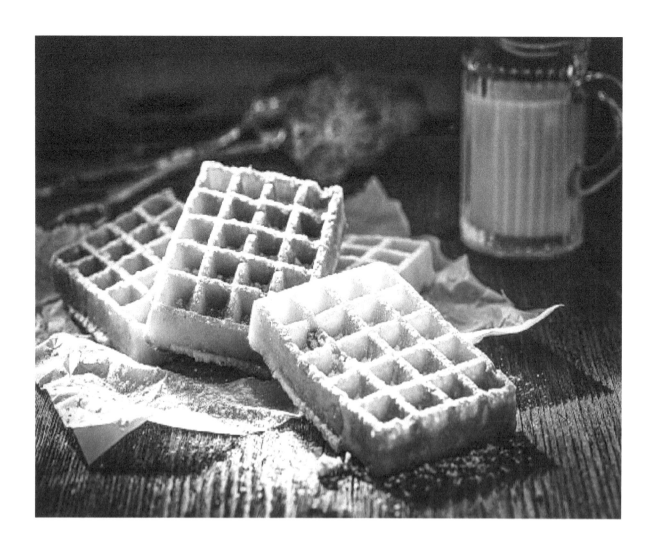

POWER PROTEIN WAFFLES

Who said waffles are unhealthy? My waffle recipes are packed full of protein and without the guilt on the side!

Nutritional value

Calories per serving: 314
Protein: 37g
Carbs: 28g
Fat: 5g

Ingredients

• 4 eggs whites
• 1 scoop of vanilla protein powder
• 40g of rolled oats
• 1 tsp of baking powder
• ½ tsp of stevia

How to make:

1. Add all the ingredients into a blender and blend.
2. Add the mixture to a waffle iron and bake.

SCRAMBLED EGGS WITH SPINACH

Tasty, quick and easy breakfast packed full of protein

Nutritional value

(Serves 2)
Calories per serving: 282
Protein: 23g
Carbs: 15g
Fat: 15g

Ingredients

- 3 eggs
- 5 egg whites
- 1 cup of baby spinach
- 50g of grated low fat cheese
- Handful of chopped onion
- Handful of chopped red peppers
- 1 tsp of olive oil

How to make:

1. Spray pan with cooking spray and place over medium/high heat.
2. Add the chopped onions, chopped red peppers and cook until soft.
3. Add the egg and egg whites to the pan with the veggies with 1tsp of olive oil and scramble until the eggs become firm.
4. Sprinkle the baby spinach leaves and cheese over the eggs.
5. Plate up and serve scrambled eggs.
6. Add salt and pepper as required.

CHAPTER 5: CHICKEN AND POULTRY

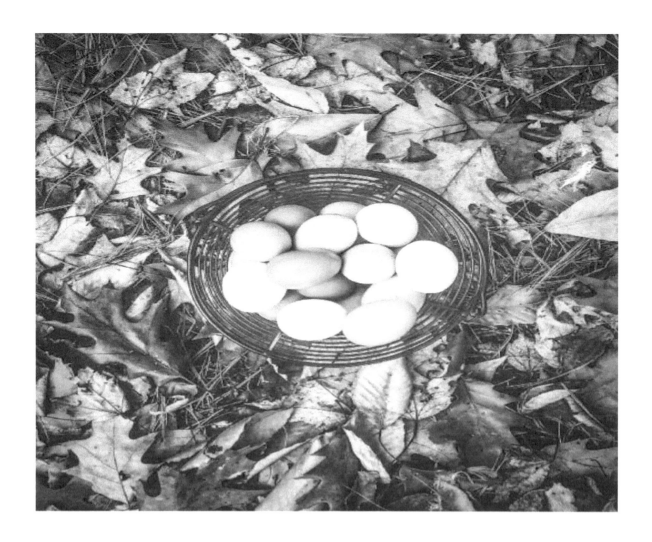

CHICKEN AND POULTRY

Chicken breast and eggs. The first things you might be mistaken to think you have to subject yourself to for breakfast, lunch and dinner for the rest of your muscle-building life. But there is so much more out there within the chicken and poultry meal options. We all know chicken is great – it's low in fat and high in protein and we all know it's tasty so read on and find out how chicken and other poultry members can be exciting and effective in your meal-plan diary.

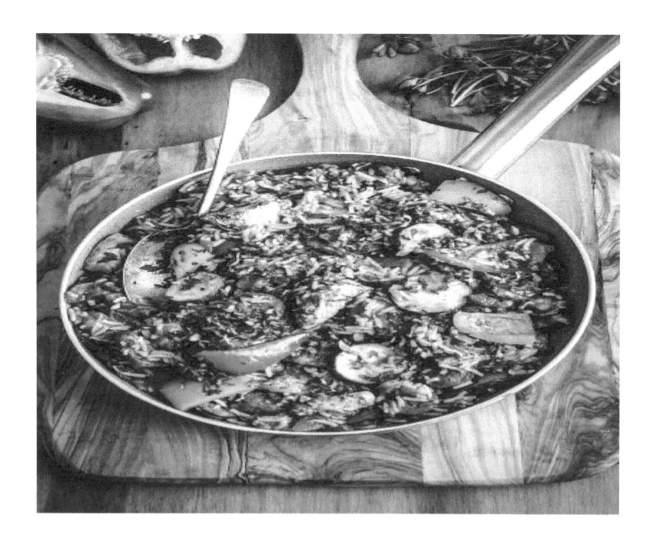

BRAWNY CHICKEN & CHORIZO JAMBALAYA

A very tasty muscle-building recipe, inspired by Cajun cuisine. Contains a good helping of protein and slow releasing carbs to keep you burning fat and building muscle.

Nutritional value

(Serves 4)
Calories per serving: 286
Protein: 30g
Carbs: 61g
Fat: 14g

Ingredients

- 2 chopped chicken breasts
- 1 chopped onion
- 1 chopped red pepper
- 2 crushed garlic cloves
- 100g chorizo, sliced
- 1 tbsp Cajun seasoning
- 250g brown rice
- 1 tbsp olive oil
- 350g of tinned chopped tomatoes
- 350ml chicken stock

How to make:

1. Grab a large pan and add the olive oil and heat on a medium heat.
2. Add the chicken and brown for around 8 minutes. Place to one side.
3. Add the onion to the pan and fry until tender. Get the garlic, chorizo, Cajun seasoning and red pepper and add to the pan and cook for around 5 minutes.
4. Add the brown rice along with the chopped tomatoes, chicken and chicken stock to the pan. Cover the pan and let simmer for around 25 minutes or until the rice is soft.

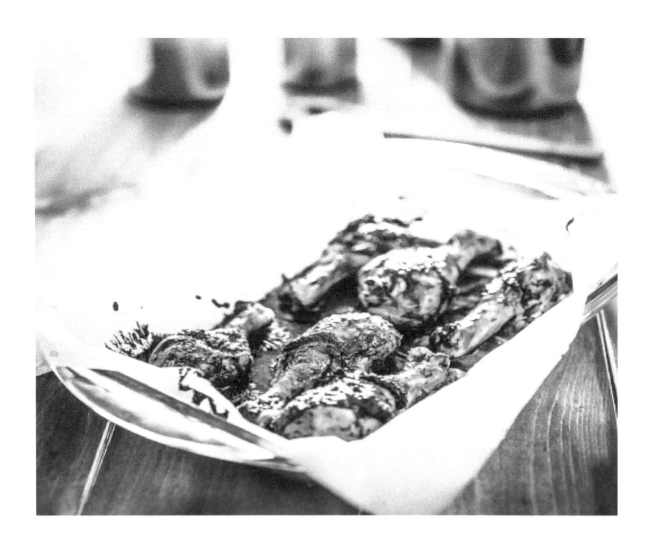

ANABOLIC JERK CHICKEN AND BROWN RICE

Add a little spice to your life with this traditional Caribbean dish. Packed full of protein and slow releasing carbohydrates to keep to you growing!

Nutritional value

Calories per serving: 516
Protein: 32g
Carbs: 76g
Fat: 33g

Ingredients

- 100g of chicken thighs or breast
- ½ tsp of ground allspice
- ½ tsp of black pepper
- ½ tsp of nutmeg
- ½ tsp of cinnamon
- ½ tsp of sage
- ½ tsp of dried thyme
- 1 clove of garlic
- ½ tsp of dried thyme
- 1 chopped onion
- 2 chopped and deseeded scotch bonnet chillies
- ½ chopped red pepper
- 60g of brown rice
- 1 tsp of olive oil

How to make:

1. To make the jerk paste, add the allspice, nutmeg, sage, cinnamon, dried thyme, garlic, red pepper, black pepper, onion, olive oil and scotch bonnet chillies to the blender and blend until it's a puree.
2. Rub the paste over the chicken breasts and leave them for at least one hour to marinade.
3. Add the chicken breasts to the grill and grill them for roughly 10-12

minutes per side or until they are cooked through. Put to one side once cooked.

4. Meanwhile add 300ml of cold water to a pot and heat until the water is boiling. Once boiling, add the rice and leave for 20 minutes.

5. Drain the rice and serve with the chicken.

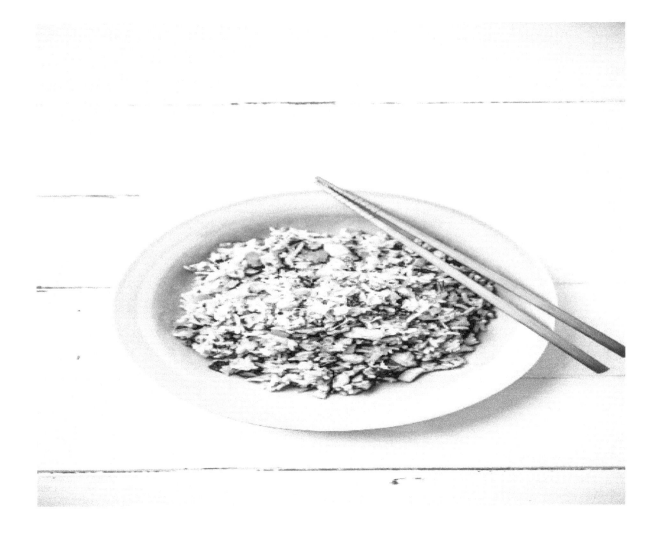

LAZY CHICKEN AND EGG STIR FRY

This meal is quick to prepare and contains two great protein sources to build muscle and burn fat.

Nutritional value

Calories per serving: 409
Protein: 46g
Carbs: 89g
Fat: 20g

Ingredients

- 100g of chopped chicken breast
- 2 eggs
- 100g of brown rice
- 2 tsp of chinese five spice
- 100g of mixed frozen veg

How to make:

1. Add 300ml of cold water to a pot and heat until the water is boiling. Once boiling, add the rice and leave for 20 minutes. Drain the rice and place to one side.
2. Heat a pan on a medium heat and add the chopped chicken and spices.
3. Stir-fry for roughly 5 minutes.
4. While the chicken is cooking, boil or steam the frozen veg for 5 minutes until cooked and beat the eggs in a separate bowl.
5. Add the rice and beaten eggs to the pan with the chicken and stir until the eggs start to scramble 3-4 minutes.
6. Finally add the veg to the pan and stir for a further

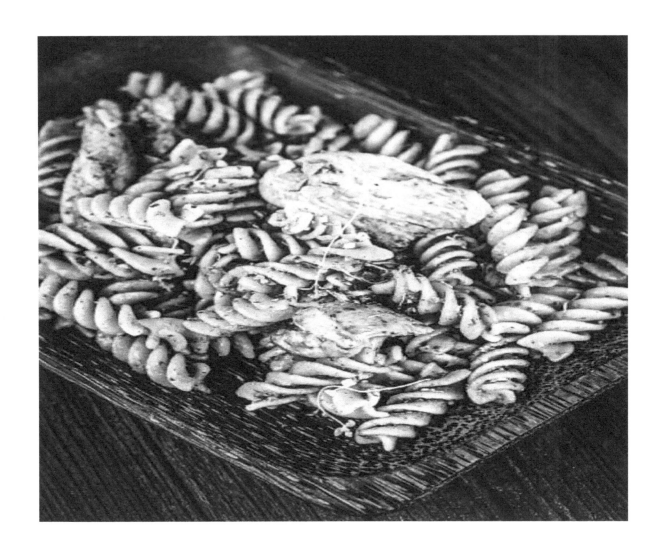

POWER PESTO CHICKEN PASTA

Great protein packed pasta dish to mix things up!

Nutritional value

(Serves 2)
Calories per serving: 550
Protein: 25g
Carbs: 30g
Fat: 19g

Ingredients

- 200g of chopped grilled chicken breast
- 100g of whole-wheat pasta
- 1 tbsp of pesto
- A pinch of black pepper
- Handful of basil
- Handful of spinach
- Handful of rocket
- Handful of pine nuts
- Handful of diced tomatoes
- 2 tbsp of olive oil

How to make:

1. Heat a large pan of water on high until it boils.
2. Add the whole-wheat pasta and leave until the water returns to boiling point.
3. Reduce the heat until the water simmers. Leave the whole-wheat pasta to cook for around 10 minutes.
4. Get a bowl and add the pesto, olive oil and black pepper and mix together.
5. Add the chopped chicken breast, pine nuts, tomatoes and herbs to the mixture.
6. Drain the pasta and fold the mix into the pan until the pasta is

covered.

MUSCLE MOROCCAN CHICKEN CASSEROLE

A classic Moroccan casserole packed with lots of protein, high in flavour and also very low in fat.

Nutritional value

(Serves 4)
Calories per serving: 404
Protein: 47g
Carbs: 37g
Fat: 8g

Ingredients

- 4 chicken breasts
- 1 tsp of ground cumin
- 1 tsp of paprika
- 1 tbsp of olive oil
- 1 chopped onion
- 350g of canned chopped tomatoes
- 2 tbsp harissa paste
- 1 tbsp honey
- 2 medium thickly sliced courgettes
- 400g of drained and rinsed chickpeas
- A pinch of salt and pepper

How to make:

1. Sprinkle salt, pepper, paprika and the ground cumin over the chicken breasts.
2. Then grab a large pan and add the olive oil and heat on a medium heat.
3. Add the chicken and onions to the pan and cook the chicken for roughly four minutes per side.
4. Pour the chopped tomatoes into the pan along with 200ml of water and add the honey, harissa, courgettes and chickpeas and stir the

ingredients together.

5. Bring the mix to a simmer and then leave to cook for around 15 minutes.

6. Plate up and serve.

SPICY CHICKEN TRAY-BAKE

A very simple to make chicken recipe that tastes great and contains all the necessary muscle building nutrients.

Nutritional value

(Serves 4)
Calories per serving: 276
Protein: 40g
Carbs: 14g
Fat: 7g

Ingredients

- 4 skinless chicken breasts
- 3 tbsp harissa paste
- 250g of low-fat natural yogurt
- 1 small, chopped and peeled butternut squash
- 2 chopped red onions
- 1 tbsp olive oil

How to make:

1. Pre-heat oven (375°F/190 °C/Gas Mark 5).
2. Add 3 tbsp of yogurt and 2 tbsp of the harissa to a bowl and mix together. Coat the chicken breast with the mixture and leave to one side.
3. Add the onions, chopped butternut squash, 1 tbsp of harissa and 2 tbsp of olive oil to a tray and place in the oven and cook for around 10 minutes. Take the tray out of the oven and add the chicken breast to the tray. Place back in the oven and cook for around 20 minutes until the chicken is cooked right through.
4. Plate up and serve with the leftover yogurt.

HEALTHY TURKEY BURGERS

Get your burger fix with this healthy turkey alternative.

Nutritional value

(Serves 4)
Calories per serving: 362
Protein: 38g
Carbs: 39g
Fat: 7g

Ingredients

• 500g of mince turkey
• 1 onion, finely chopped
• 1 chopped romaine lettuce
• 4 wholemeal buns
• 2 diced tomatoes
• 1 crushed garlic clove
• 1 lemon
• 3 tbsp grated parmesan
• Chopped parsley
• 3 tbsp low-fat Greek yogurt

How to make:

1. Pre-heat oven (375°F/190 °C/Gas Mark 5).
2. In a bowl, add the crushed garlic, 2 tbsp of parmesan and parsley.
3. Cut the lemon in half and squeeze the lemon juice over the ingredients. Mix all the ingredients together.
4. Add the ingredients to the minced turkey along with the onion and mix them together.
5. Using your hands, mould the mince mixture into 4 burgers and place on a tray and then cook for around 20 minutes or until the burgers have cooked right through.
6. While the burgers are cooking, cut open the whole-wheat buns and

mix the yogurt with the lettuce. Add the burgers to the buns along with the yogurt-lettuce mixture and tomatoes.

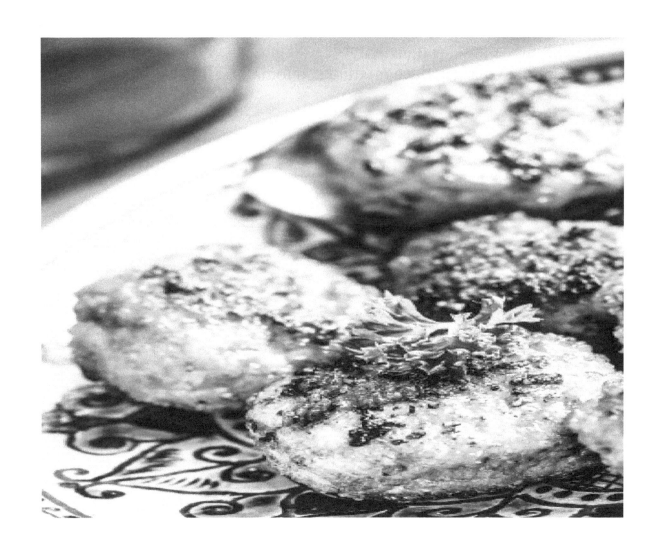

TURKEY MEATBALL FIESTA

Healthy turkey meatballs with added oats to keep you building muscle and burning fat.

Nutritional value

(Serves 4)
Calories per serving: 315
Protein: 35g
Carbs: 23g
Fat: 10g

Ingredients

- 500g of turkey mince
- 50g rolled porridge oats
- 2 chopped spring onions
- 1 tsp ground cumin
- 1 tsp coriander
- Handful of chopped coriander
- 1 tsp olive oil
- 1 chopped red onion
- 2 chopped garlic cloves
- 1 large chopped yellow pepper
- 3 tsp chipotle chilli paste
- 300ml chicken stock
- 400g of canned chopped tomatoes
- 400g of drained black beans
- 1 avocado, stoned, peeled and chopped

How to make:

1. Add the mince to a bowl with the oats, chopped spring onions, spices and coriander and mix together.
2. Mould the mince mixture into 12 small 'meatballs' using your hands.

3. Add some olive oil to the pan on a medium heat; add the meatballs and cook them until golden.
4. Take them from the pan and leave to one side.
5. Add the onion, chopped pepper and chopped garlic to the pan and cook until tender.
6. Add the chilli paste and ground cumin and chicken stock to the pan and stir well. Then add the meatballs back into the pan.
7. Cover and cook on a low/medium heat for around 10 minutes.
8. Add the tomatoes and black beans to the pan and cook uncovered for around 2-3 minutes.
9. Serve with the chopped avocado and coriander.

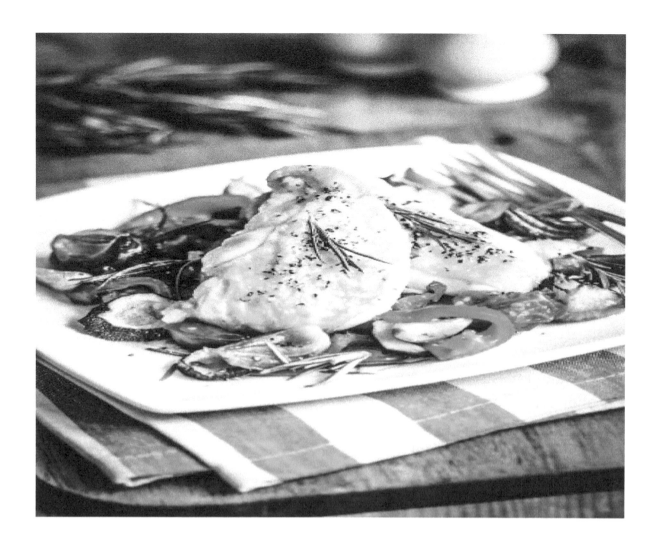

ANABOLIC RATATOUILLE CHICKEN

A tasty low-carb chicken recipe to keep you building muscle and burning fat.

Nutritional value

(Serves 4)
Calories per serving: 324
Protein: 38g
Carbs: 10g
Fat: 15g

Ingredients

- 4 chicken breasts
- 1 chopped onion,
- 2 chopped red peppers
- 1 courgette, cut into chunks
- 1 small aubergine, cut into chunks
- 4 chopped tomatoes
- 4 tbsp of olive oil
- A pinch of salt and pepper

How to make:

1. Pre-heat oven (375°F/190 °C/Gas Mark 5).
2. Add all the vegetables and the tomatoes to a tray and drizzle with 3 tbsp. olive oil.
3. Place the chicken breasts over the vegetables and season with the remaining tbsp of olive oil and some salt and pepper.
4. Place the tray in the oven and cook for around 30 minutes.
5. Plate up and serve

BRAWNY CHICKEN CHASSEUR

A classic and tasty chicken dish, packed with protein and low in carbs.

Nutritional value

(Serves 4)
Calories per serving: 242
Protein: 50g
Carbs: 5g
Fat: 3g

Ingredients

- 8 chopped rashers of turkey bacon
- 4 chopped chicken breasts
- 200g of baby mushrooms
- 1 tbsp plain flour
- 400g of canned chopped tomatoes
- 1 beef stock cube
- 1 tbsp Worcestershire sauce
- Handful of chopped parsley
- 1 tbsp olive oil

How to make:

1. Heat the olive oil on a medium heat in a shallow saucepan and add the turkey bacon and cook for 4-5 minutes until it starts to brown.
2. Add the chopped chicken breasts and cook for around 5 minutes until golden. Increase the heat to high and add the baby mushrooms for 2 minutes. Add the flour and stir in until a paste starts to form.
3. Add the canned chopped tomatoes and beef stock cube to the saucepan and cook for around 10 minutes.
4. Then add the parsley and Worcestershire sauce to the pan, stir in and then serve.

AESTHETIC TOMATO AND OLIVE PAN-FRIED CHICKEN

A tasty chicken dish, sure to satisfy your hunger and nutritional needs.

Nutritional value

(Serves 2)
Calories per serving: 334
Protein: 39g
Carbs: 8g
Fat: 19g

Ingredients

- 2 chicken breasts
- 1 chopped onion,
- 2 chopped garlic cloves
- 400g of canned chopped tomatoes
- 1 tbsp balsamic vinegar
- 6 chopped green olives
- 300ml chicken stock
- 2 tbsp olive oil
- Handful of basil leaves
- A pinch of salt and pepper

How to make:

1. Heat olive oil on a medium heat in a pan.
2. Sprinkle some salt and pepper over the chicken and then place the chicken in the pan and cook for roughly 10 minutes, or until the chicken has cooked right through..
3. Add the onion to the pan and turn the chicken over and cook for another 4 – 5 minutes. Remove the chicken from the pan and place to one side.
4. Add the garlic to the pan and continue to cook the onions until tender.
5. Add the chopped tomatoes, olives, chicken stock and balsamic

vinegar to the pan with most of the basil leaves and turn down the heat, simmering for around 8 minutes.

6. Place the chicken back into the pan, cover and simmer for a further 5 minutes

7. Plate up and serve with the remaining basil as a garnish.

CHICKEN BRAWN BURGER

Another great healthy burger alternative! Quick and easy to make if you're strapped for time. Contains a good helping of protein to keep you anabolic.

Nutritional value

Calories per serving: 458
Protein: 50g
Carbs: 38g
Fat: 12g

Ingredients

- 1 chicken breast
- 1 tbsp low fat mayonnaise
- 1 chopped red onion
- 1 chopped lettuce
- 1 slice of low-fat cheddar
- 1 whole wheat burger bun
- 1 tsp of chopped jalapeno slices
- 1 tsp olive oil

How to make:

1. Heat olive oil on a medium heat in a griddle pan.
2. Cover the chicken breast with some salt and pepper and add to the pan and cook for around 5 minutes. Turn it over and cook for a further 5 minutes.
3. Add the slice of cheddar to the top of the chicken. Cook chicken for another 8 minutes or until chicken is cooked right through.
4. Remove chicken from pan and place to one side.
5. Cut open the roll and add the chicken, onions, mayonnaise, lettuce and chopped jalapeno

TASTY TURKEY BAGEL

A great recipe, ideal for lunch or post-workout! Contains lots of protein to keep you growing.

Nutritional value

Calories per serving: 336
Protein: 21g
Carbs: 64g
Fat: 1g

Ingredients

- 2 thick deli turkey breast slices (cooked)
- 1 whole-wheat bagel
- Handful of baby spinach
- Handful of rocket
- 1 chopped tomato
- ¼ sliced cucumber

How to make:

1. Cut the whole-wheat bagel in half and then add each half to the toaster.
2. Add the turkey breast, chopped tomato, cucumber, spinach and rocket to the bagel.
3. Serve on the go or at home!

DICED CHICKEN WITH EGG NOODLES

Go ahead and mix things up with this tasty recipe. Contains the right amount of protein, carbs and fats to meet your goals.

Nutritional value

(Serves 2)
Calories per serving: 322
Protein: 30g
Carbs: 31g
Fat: 8g

Ingredients

- 150g of chopped chicken breast
- 50g of whole-wheat noodles
- 1 grated carrot
- 2 tbsp of fresh orange juice
- 1 tsp of sesame seeds
- 3 tsp of soy sauce
- 2 tsp of rapeseed oil
- 1 chopped ginger
- 100g of sugar snap peas

How to make:

1. Heat 1 tsp rapeseed oil on a medium heat in pan.
2. Cook the chopped chicken breast for about 10-15 minutes or until cooked through.
3. While cooking the chicken, place the noodles in a pot of boiling water for about 5 minutes.
4. In a bowl, mix together the ginger, sesame seeds, soy sauce, 1 tsp rapeseed oil and orange juice.

HONEY GLAZED GROWTH CHICKEN

Mix things up with this sweet and tempting chicken recipe.

Nutritional value

(Serves 2)
Calories per serving: 195
Protein: 37g
Carbs: 9g
Fat: 2g

Ingredients

- 2 chicken breasts with skin on
- ½ lemon
- 1 tbsp honey
- 1 tbsp dark soy sauce
- A pinch of salt and pepper

How to make:

1. Pre-heat oven (375°F/190 °C/Gas Mark 5).
2. Place the chicken breast on a baking dish and add a sprinkle of salt and pepper.
3. Get a bowl and squeeze the lemon juice in and add the honey and soy sauce. Mix the ingredients together and cover the chicken breasts with it.
4. Place the squeezed lemon in between the chicken breasts and place the dish into the oven and cook for around 30 minutes on until fully cooked through.

MIGHTY MEXICAN CHICKEN STEW

Spice things up with this classic Mexican chicken stew. Packed full of protein from the chicken as well as the quinoa!

Nutritional value

(Serves 4)
Calories per serving: 464
Protein: 51g
Carbs: 53g
Fat: 4g

Ingredients

- 4 skinless chicken breasts
- 140g quinoa
- 400g of drained pinto beans
- 1 tbsp olive oil
- 1 chopped onion
- 2 chopped red peppers
- 3 tbsp chipotle paste
- 800g of tinned chopped tomatoes
- 2 chicken stock cubes
- Handful of chopped coriander
- 1 lime

How to make:

1. Heat olive oil on a medium heat in a deep pan and add the onion and peppers and cook for 2-3 minutes.
2. Then add the chipotle paste and the tinned chopped tomatoes.
3. Add the chicken breast and add just enough water to cover the chicken by 1cm and then bring down the heat to let the mixture simmer. Cook for around 20 minutes until the chicken is cooked right through.
4. Add boiling water to a separate saucepan along with stock cubes.

Pour in the quinoa and heat for around 12 minutes.

5. Add the pinto beans and cook for a further 3 minutes. Drain the quinoa and add in the coriander and squeeze the lime juice in - mix and place to one side.

6. Serve the chicken with the quinoa and cover with the tomato sauce from the pan.

SPICY CAJUN CHICKEN WITH GUACAMOLE

Tasty low fat, low carb chicken recipe! Contains a generous amount of protein to keep you building muscle and burning fat.

Nutritional value

(Serves 4)
Calories per serving: 190
Protein: 34g
Carbs: 2g
Fat: 5g

Ingredients

- 4 chicken breasts
- 1 tbsp paprika
- 1 tsp dried onion flakes
- ¼ tsp cayenne pepper
- 2 tsp dried thyme
- A pinch of salt and pepper
- 1 tbsp olive oil
- 200g of guacamole

How to make:

1. Get a bowl and add the cayenne pepper, dried thyme, paprika, salt, pepper and onion flakes and mix together.
2. Get the chicken and cut two deep scores on each breast. Rub the oil onto the chicken then cover the breasts with the spices.
3. Add the chicken to the grill and cook for around 8 minutes each side or until completely cooked through.
4. Serve chicken with the guacamole

MUSCLE CHICKEN CACCIATORE

An Italian inspired, delicious, low fat, low carb chicken recipe. Contains a liberal amount of protein to keep you building muscle and burning fat.

Nutritional value

(Serves 4)
Calories per serving: 172
Protein: 33g
Carbs: 6g
Fat: 2g

Ingredients

- 4 chicken breasts
- 1 chopped onion
- 2 sliced garlic cloves
- A pinch of salt and pepper
- 1 tsp olive oil
- 400g of tinned chopped tomatoes
- 2 tbsp chopped rosemary leaves
- Handful of basil leaves

How to make:

1. Pre-Heat oven (375°F/190 °C/Gas Mark 5).
2. Heat oil in a pan on a medium heat and add the onion and garlic and cook until soft.
3. Pour in the chopped tomatoes, rosemary, salt and pepper and cook for around 15 minutes until the mixture has become thicker.
4. Spread the mixture over the chicken; place the chicken on a tray and transfer to the oven. Leave in the oven for 20 minutes until the chicken is cooked right through. Sprinkle the basil over the chicken and serve.

CHAPTER 6: RED MEAT AND PORK

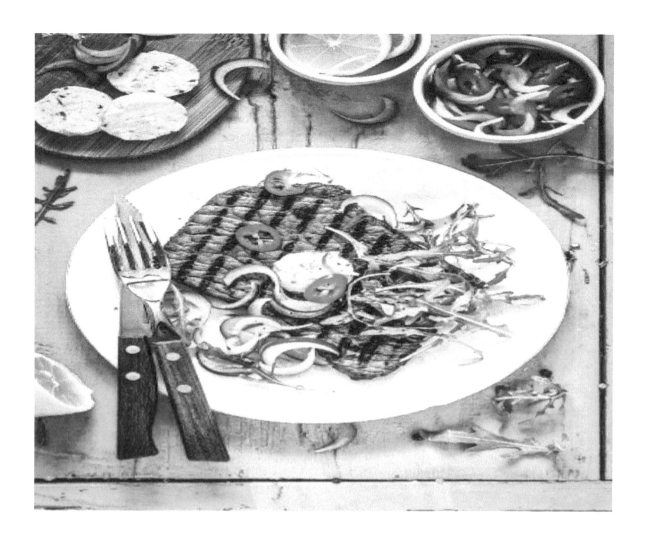

RED MEAT AND PORK

I've teamed pork with red meat because it has every bit as much macho power! Pork doesn't have to be dry and fatty it can be delicious with the recipes to follow. Red meat speaks for itself in the muscle building world – a slab of steak comes to anybody's mind when they are trying to get big! Hopefully from the next section I can provide you with alternative dishes to fill you up with iron, protein and much more!

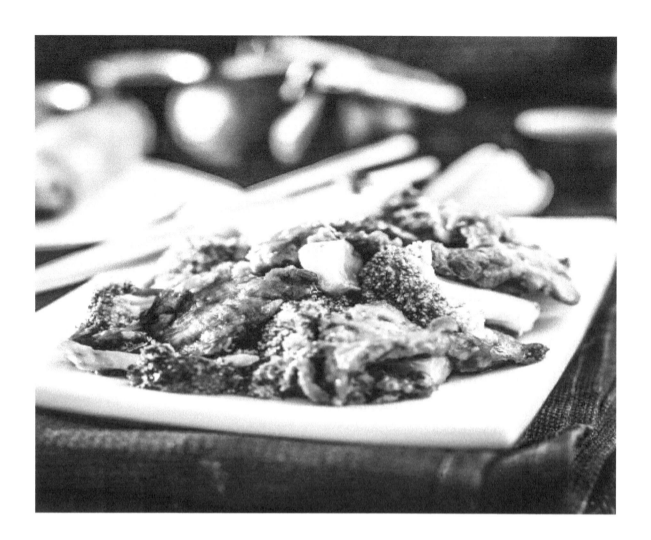

TASTY BEEF BROCCOLI STIR FRY

A very quick and easy, healthy beef stir-fry that will save you reaching out for the local Chinese delivery menu!

Nutritional value

(Serves 4)
Calories per serving: 277
Protein: 30g
Carbs: 7g
Fat: 14g

Ingredients

• 400g of diced frying beef steaks
• 1 head of broccoli, broken into florets
• 4 chopped celery sticks
• Handful of sweet corn
• 150ml beef stock
• 2 tbsp of horseradish sauce
• 1 tbsp of olive oil
• A pinch of salt and pepper

How to make:

1. Heat the olive oil on a medium/high heat in a frying pan.
2. Add some salt and pepper to the beefsteaks and place in the frying pan.
3. Stir-fry for 2 minutes until the beef is browned then remove and set aside.
4. Add the broccoli and chopped celery to the pan and fry for a further 2 minutes.
5. Add the beef stock to the pan, then cover. Reduce the heat and let the veg simmer for 2 minutes.
6. Place the steak back in the pan and mix with the other vegetables for another minute.

7. Plate up and serve with the horseradish sauce.

ANABOLIC PORK SOUP

This soup is quick to prepare and full of protein to build muscle and burn fat.

Nutritional value

(Serves 4)
Calories per serving: 297
Protein: 21g
Carbs: 13g
Fat: 17g

Ingredients

- 400g diced pork steaks
- 600ml chicken stock
- 1 tbsp soy sauce
- 2 tsp Chinese five-spice powder
- 25 ginger finely chopped
- 200g pack of baby spinach
- 1 tsp of chopped red chilli,
- 200g of rice noodles
- Handful of chopped spring onions

How to make:

1. Get a large saucepan and add all the ingredients except for the spring onions and noodles. Cover the pan and bring to a simmer on a medium heat.
2. Without letting the ingredients boil, leave to cook for around 8-10 minutes.
3. While cooking the pork, place the rice noodles in a pot of boiling water for about 5 minutes and then drain.
4. Drain and place the noodles in a bowl and add the pork and greens over the noodles. Sprinkle the spring onions over the dish and serve.

POWER PORK FRUIT TRAY

This dish is absolutely delicious and one of my favourite pork recipes. Contains a good helping of protein and is low on carbs for those of you who are shredding!

Nutritional value

(Serves 4)
Calories per serving: 335
Protein: 42g
Carbs: 12g
Fat: 14g

Ingredients

- 4 pork steaks
- 1 tbsp olive oil
- 2 diced red onions
- 2 chopped large pears
- 3 sprigs of rosemary
- 50g diced blue cheese
- 1 diced courgette
- A pinch of salt and pepper
- Handful of pine nuts

How to make:

1. Get a large pan and heat the olive oil on a medium heat.
2. Add the courgette, red onions, chopped pears, salt and pepper.
3. Fry for around 6 minutes until the veg starts to caramelise.
4. Pre-heat the Grill.
5. Get a cooking tray and transfer the ingredients along with the rosemary sprigs to the tray. Sprinkle some salt and pepper over the pork steaks and place them in the tray.
6. Place the tray in the oven and grill for around 10-15 minutes or until cooked right through, turning the pork steaks half way through. Add

the cheese and pine nuts and let the cheese melt for a further 4-5 minutes.

7. Plate up and serve.

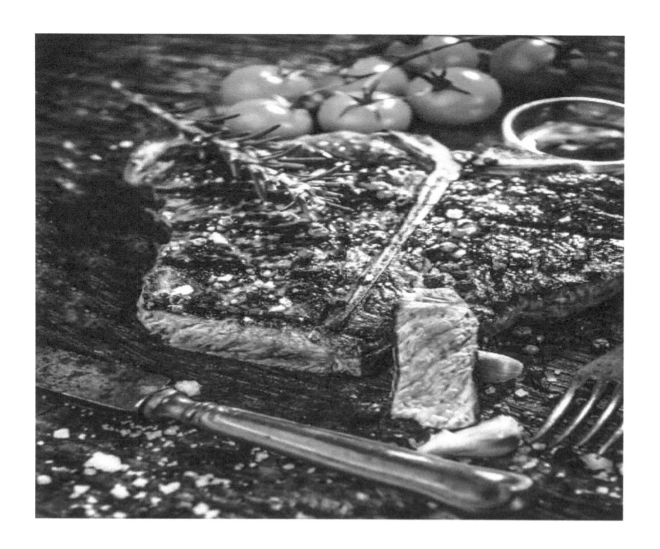

MUSCLE BUILDING STEAK & SWEET POTATO FRIES

A great, healthy alternative to regular steak and chips! Contains a good helping of protein and slow releasing carbs.

Nutritional value

(Serves 4)
Calories per serving: 418
Protein: 29g
Carbs: 39g
Fat: 15g

Ingredients

- 100g of sirloin steak
- 200g of sweet potatoes cut into chips
- 1 tbsp olive oil
- 1 chopped red onion
- 1 bag of pre-washed salad
- 1 tbsp of balsamic vinegar
- A pinch of black pepper

How to make:

1. Pre-Heat oven (375°F/190 °C/Gas Mark 5).
2. Get a baking tray, spread the chips out and bake for around 25 minutes.
3. While the chips are cooking, get a large frying pan and heat the olive oil on a medium heat.
4. Pepper the steaks and add to the pan. Fry the steaks for 6 minutes in total, turning the steaks once halfway through.
5. Take the steak and leave to cool.
6. Get a large bowl and add the salad and chopped onion. Drizzle with the vinegar and serve with the potatoes and steak.

ORIENTAL BEEF MUSCLE STIR-FRY

Great beef recipe, packed with loads of protein to keep you growing and burning fat.

Nutritional value

(Serves 4)
Calories per serving: 349
Protein: 34g
Carbs: 26g
Fat: 14g

Ingredients

- 500g of diced beef rump
- 1 tsp Chinese five-spice powder
- 300g of egg noodles
- 1 large chopped red chilli
- 1 chopped garlic clove
- 1 chopped thumb-size piece of ginger
- 1 stick lemongrass
- 2 tbsp of olive oil
- 100g sugar snap peas
- 8 baby corns, sliced diagonally
- 6 chopped spring onions
- ½ lime
- 2 tbsp soy sauce
- 1 tbsp fish sauce
- 2 tbsp roasted peanuts
- Handful of chopped coriander, to serve

How to make:

1. Get a bowl and add the beef and five-spice and leave to marinade. Place the egg noodles in a pot of boiling water for about 5 minutes, drain and then place to one side.

2. Mix together the chopped chilli, ginger, garlic and lemongrass in a bowl.
3. Add 1 tbsp of olive oil to a wok and heat on a medium heat. Add the ginger mixture into the wok and fry for 1 minute. Turn up the heat and add 1 more tbsp of olive oil to the wok and add the beef and fry until browned.
4. Add the sugar snaps, spring onions and baby corn to the wok and continue to stir-fry for around a minute before adding the egg noodles and mix together. Turn off the heat and add the soy sauce, fish sauces and squeezed lime juice.
5. Place in a bowl and add the peanuts and chopped coriander to serve.

BULK-UP LAMB CURRY & PEANUT STEW

This absolutely delicious curry is packed full of flavour and has a hefty dose of protein to boot.

Nutritional value

(Serves 4)
Calories per serving: 600
Protein: 44g
Carbs: 38g
Fat: 46g

Ingredients

- 50g chopped peanuts
- 400ml canned coconut cream
- 4 tbsp massaman curry paste
- 600g diced lamb steak (or beef)
- 450g chopped white potatoes
- 1 chopped onion
- 1 cinnamon stick
- 1 tbsp tamarind paste
- 1 tbsp fish sauce
- 1 sliced red chilli

How to make:

1. Pre-heat oven (375°F/190 °C/Gas Mark 5).
2. Get a large casserole dish and place on the gas/electric hob on a medium heat.
3. Add 2 tbsp of coconut cream and the curry paste and fry for around a minute before adding the diced lamb. Stir in and brown. Add the rest of the coconut cream with a cup of water as well as the potatoes, onions, cinnamon stick, tamarind, fish sauce and peanuts.
4. Reduce heat to a simmer, cover the casserole, transfer to the oven and cook for 2 hours until the lamb is soft and tender.

5. Add the sliced chilli to the top and serve.

BRAWNY BEEF FAJITAS

Quick and easy beef recipe, perfect for lunch and packed with loads of protein to keep you growing and burning fat.

Nutritional value

Calories per serving: 358
Protein: 28g
Carbs: 40g
Fat: 10g

Ingredients

- 100g of diced lean steak
- 1 chopped red onion
- 1 chopped red pepper
- 1 wholegrain fajita wrap
- 2 tbsp of sweet chilli sauce

How to make:

1. Add the diced steak, chopped onion, red pepper and 1 tbsp of chilli sauce to a pan and stir fry for around 4 – 5 minutes on a medium to high heat.
2. Place the wrap in the microwave for 30 seconds or under a grill for the same amount of time.
3. Add the steak mix to the fajita, along with one more tbsp of sweet chilli sauce.
4. Roll up and enjoy!

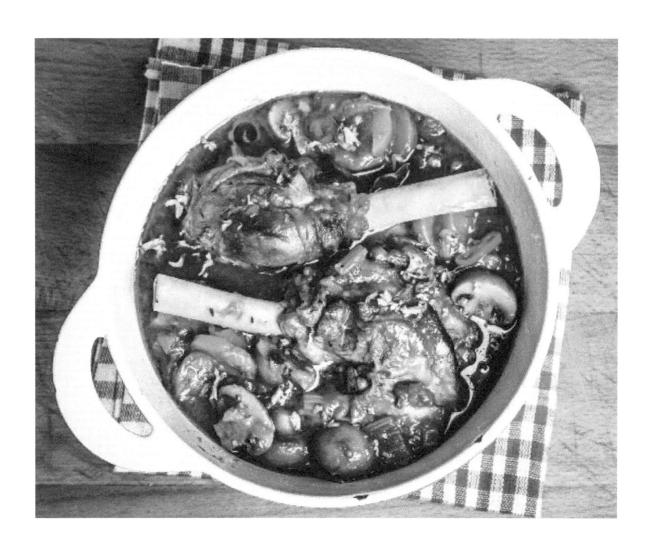

MIGHTY LAMB CASSEROLE

This meal is absolutely delicious and easy to make!

Nutritional value

(Serves 2)
Calories per serving: 380
Protein: 35g
Carbs: 33g
Fat: 9g

Ingredients

- 1 tbsp of olive oil
- 2 cubed lamb fillets
- 1 chopped onion
- 2 chopped carrots, thickly sliced
- Handful of kale
- 400ml of chicken stock
- 1 tsp dried rosemary
- 1 tsp of chopped parsley
- 400g of rinsed and drained cannellini beans

How to make:

1. Get a large casserole dish and heat the olive oil on a medium heat.
2. Add the lamb to the casserole dish and cook for 5 minutes until browned, then add the chopped onion and carrots. Leave to cook for another 5 minutes until the vegetables begin to soften.
3. Add the chicken stock, kale and rosemary. Then cover the casserole, leave to simmer on a low heat for 1-1.5 hours until the lamb is tender and fully cooked through.
4. Add the cannellini beans 15 minutes before the end of the cooking time.
5. Plate up and serve with the chopped parsley to garnish.

STEAK & CHEESE MUSCLE CLUB

An extremely healthy homemade sandwich with a generous amount of protein to ensure you are building muscle and burning fat.

Nutritional value

(Serves 2)
Calories per serving: 336
Protein: 32g
Carbs: 27g
Fat: 11g

Ingredients

- 1 250g sirloin steak
- 2 whole-meal bread rolls
- 1 tsp olive oil
- 1 tsp Dijon mustard
- Handful of rocket
- 30g Stilton cheese
- 1 tsp of balsamic vinegar
- A pinch of salt and pepper

How to make:

1. Heat up a griddle pan on a high heat until very hot. Drizzle the olive oil over the steak over both sides of the steak. Sprinkle some salt and pepper over it and place the steak in the pan and fry for 3 minutes on each side. Place the steak to one side and leave to rest for a minute.
2. Cut in half to form two slices of steak.
3. Cut the whole-wheat rolls in half and place toast. Once done, add the mustard and rocket to the roll and place 1 half of the steak on top. Add balsamic vinegar and the cheese to the top and then make the sandwich.
4. Repeat steps with the other roll.

MASS GAINING LAMB FLATBREAD

A tasty and healthy homemade flatbread with a Moroccan twist, including a generous amount of protein to fuel you and your muscles!

Nutritional value

(Serves 4)
Calories per serving: 391
Protein: 29g
Carbs: 34g
Fat: 17g

Ingredients

• 2 200g lamb leg steaks
• 1 tbsp harissa
• 4 whole meal flatbreads
• 4 tbsp of organic houmous
• Handful of baby spinach
• Handful of watercress
• A pinch of salt and pepper

How to make:

1. Preheat the grill.
2. Sprinkle harissa, salt and pepper over the lamb.
3. Place lamb on a baking tray and grill for 4 minutes before turning the lamb over and cooking for a further 4 minutes. Take the tray out of the grill and leave to one side.
4. Place the flatbreads under the grill for around 1 – 2 minutes before removing and spreading on the houmous.
5. Cut the lamb into thin strips and place over the flat bread.

SUPER STEAK WITH SPICY RICE & BEANS

The perfect steak…
Nutritional value
(Serves 2)
Calories per serving: 650
Protein: 48g
Carbs: 60g
Fat: 26g

Ingredients

- 2 250g sirloin steaks
- 4 tsp olive oil
- 1 small onion, sliced
- 100g brown long-grain rice
- 1½tsp fajita seasoning
- 1 can of drained kidney beans
- Handful of chopped coriander leaves
- 2 tbsp tomato salsa, to serve

How to make:

1. Pour 3 tsp of oil into a deep saucepan on a medium heat and add the onion. Fry the onion for around 4 minutes.
2. Then add ½ the fajita seasoning and long grain rice. Cook for 1 minute. Add 300ml of boiling water to the saucepan and stir in. Cover the saucepan and let simmer for 20 minutes until the water has been absorbed and the rice is fluffy. Add the kidney beans and keep the pan warm.
3. While the rice is cooking, sprinkle salt and pepper over the steak as well as ½ fajita seasoning. Pre-heat a griddle pan on a high heat, add the steaks and cook for 8 minutes in total, turning the steaks half way through.
4. Add the rice to a bowl and mix in the coriander. Add a tbsp of tomato salsa to each of the steaks and serve.

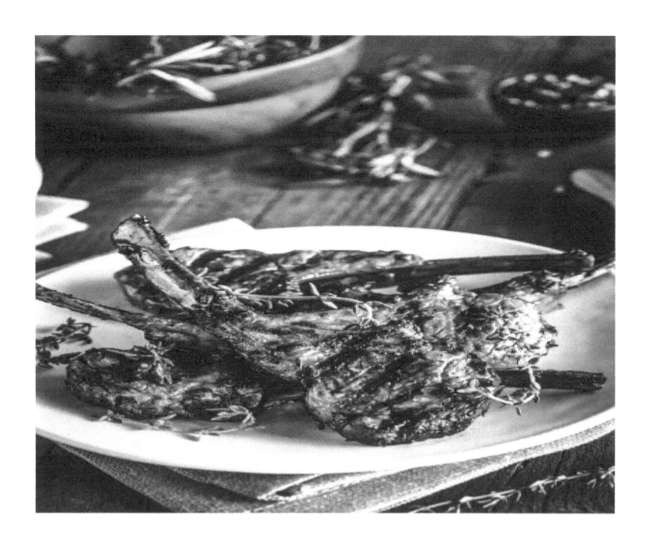

MUSCLE MINT LAMB STEAKS

Delicious recipe with over 40g of protein to keep you building muscle and burning fat!

Nutritional value

(Serves 2)
Calories per serving: 367
Protein: 41g
Carbs: 2g
Fat: 22g

Ingredients

• 4 200g lamb leg steaks
• 2 tbsp olive oil
• 2 chopped garlic cloves
• 1 tbsp balsamic vinegar
• Handful of chopped mint leaves

How to make:

1. Get a bowl and add the mint, vinegar and garlic and mix together.
2. Add the lamb to the bowl and leave to marinade for at least 30 minutes.
3. Pre-heat a griddle pan on a medium to high heat and cook the lamb for 4 minutes each side or until cooked through.
4. Serve alone or with your choice of salad for a delicious accompaniment.

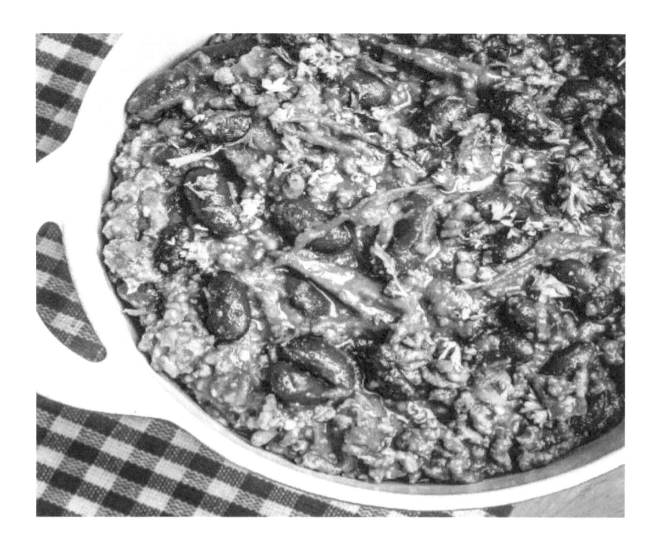

SUPER LAMB STEAKS WITH MEDITERRANEAN VEG

A mediterranean twist on a lamb dish! A very quick and easy, healthy lamb recipe to keep you going for longer…

Nutritional value

(Serves 2)
Calories per serving: 308
Protein: 34g
Carbs: 15g
Fat: 14g

Ingredients

- 2 200g lamb leg/breast steaks
- 2 chopped courgettes
- 2 tbsp olive oil
- Handful of rocket
- 2 garlic cloves, chopped
- 8 halved baby cherry tomatoes
- Handful of chopped coriander

How to make:

1. Preheat the grill.
2. Add the oil to a pan and heat on a medium heat.
3. Throw in the courgettes, tomatoes and garlic and fry until courgettes and tomatoes are soft.
4. Add the rocket and coriander and stir in.
5. Meanwhile, sprinkle some salt and pepper over the lamb steaks. Place the lamb on a tray and grill for 4 minutes each side.
6. Serve alongside the veg.

STRENGTH AND MASS MEATLOAF

The perfect muscle building meatloaf!

Nutritional value

(Serves 6)
Calories per serving: 410
Protein: 47g
Carbs: 15g
Fat: 19g

Ingredients

- 900g of lean ground beef
- 1 tsp olive oil
- 1 chopped red onion
- 1 tsp garlic
- 3 chopped tomatoes
- 1 whole beaten egg
- 100g of whole wheat bread crumbs
- Handful of parsley
- 20g of low fat parmesan
- 50ml of organic skim milk
- A pinch of salt and pepper
- 1 tsp oregano

How to make:

1. Preheat the oven to (400°F/200 °C/Gas Mark 6).
2. Add the oil to a pan and heat on a medium heat.
3. Cook the onions until soft but not browned. Remove the onions from the pan and let cool.
4. Get a big bowl and mix all of the ingredients together.
5. Put the meat in a big baking tray and cook on a high heat for around 30-35 minutes.
6. Serve once cooked through and piping hot.

FARLEY'S MUSCLE BUILDING CHILLI CON CARNE

Who doesn't like Chilli con carne? Well this healthy version will provide you with over 30g of protein and a smug sense of satisfaction!

Nutritional value

(Serves 4)
Calories per serving: 389
Protein: 37g
Carbs: 25g
Fat: 17g

Ingredients

- 500g lean ground beef
- 1 tbsp oil
- 1 chopped onion
- 1 chopped red pepper
- 2 crushed garlic cloves,
- 1 tsp of chilli powder
- 1 tsp paprika
- 1 tsp ground cumin
- 1 beef stock cube
- 400g of tinned chopped tomatoes
- 2 tbsp tomato purée
- 400g of dried and rinsed red kidney beans
- 100g of brown rice

How to make:

1. Get a pan and add the olive oil and heat on a medium heat.
2. Add the onions to the pan and fry until soft.
3. Then add the garlic, red pepper, chilli powder, paprika and cumin. Stir together and cook for 5 minutes.
4. Add the ground mince to the pan and cook until browned.
5. Get 300ml of hot water and add the beef stock cube to it. Add this to

the pan along with the chopped tomatoes. Also add the puree and stir in well. Bring the pan to a simmer, cover and cook for around 50 minutes. Stir occasionally.

6. After 30 minutes and while the mince is cooking, add 300ml of cold water to a separate pot and heat until the water is boiling. Once boiling, add the rice and leave for 20 minutes.

7. Once the rice is done, drain and put to one side. Add the beans to the meat mix and cook for another 10 minutes.

8. Serve the rice topped with the chilli con carne.

BRAWNY BEEF SANDWICHES

It's a hell of a lot cheaper to make your own sandwiches and a lot healthier than the shop-bought ones too. This brawny sandwich provides plenty of protein to keep you anabolic.

Nutritional value

Calories per serving: 545
Protein: 43g
Carbs: 64g
Fat: 10g

Ingredients

- 4 slices of deli beef
- 4 slices of whole-wheat bread
- 2 tsp of mustard
- Handful of baby spinach leaves
- 1/2 a sliced cucumber
- A pinch of black pepper

How to make:

1. Get 2 slices of bread.
2. Add 2 slices of deli beef, 1 tsp of mustard, ½ a sliced cucumber, spinach and a pinch of black pepper to the slice and make a sandwich.
3. Repeat the process with the rest of the ingredients.

CHAPTER 7: FISH & SEAFOOD

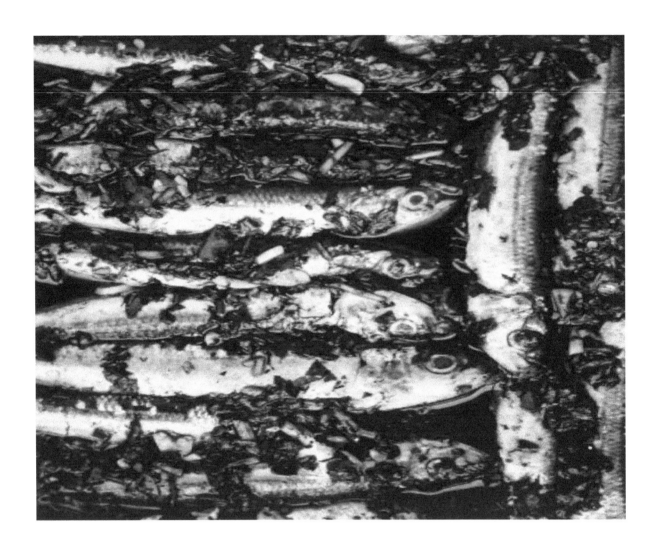

FISH & SEAFOOD

A lot of us reserve fish for the refined. Either that or we're scared of cooking it. Fish is often easier than cooking meat; it's fresh, healthy and full of omega 3. Hopefully the recipes provided in this section will either get you started with cooking up fish, or further you down the chef road you're already on. Oh, and it will mean you burn fat, build strength, and increase brain power all at the same time!

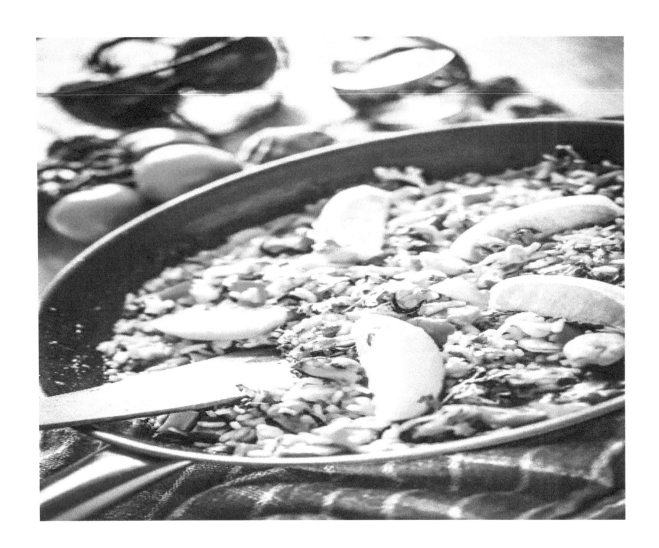

PROTEIN PACKED PAELLA

A delicious, traditional Spanish dish that's packed full over flavour and protein to ensure you continue to build muscle and burn fat.

Nutritional value

(Serves 4)
Calories per serving: 351
Protein: 21g
Carbs: 50g
Fat: 9g

Ingredients

• 200g frozen cooked prawns
• 2 diced chorizo sausages
• 1 tbsp olive oil
• 1 chopped onion
• 1 chopped garlic clove
• ½ tsp turmeric
• 600g cooked brown rice
• 100g frozen peas

How to make:

1. Heat olive oil in a pan on a high heat. Add the chorizo, onion and garlic and then fry for 2-3 minutes until soft.
2. Add the turmeric, rice, prawns and frozen peas as well as 100ml of boiling water.
3. Stir until everything is warm and the water has been absorbed.
4. Plate up and serve.

MUSCLE MACKEREL AND SPICY COUSCOUS

Mackerel is a great healthy source of protein and is also a great source of omega-3 fats.

Nutritional value

Calories per serving: 484
Protein: 26g
Carbs: 35g
Fat: 26g

Ingredients

- 150g of couscous
- 100g of pre cooked mackerel
- 1tsp of ground cumin
- 1 tsp of smoked paprika
- 1 chopped red chilli
- Pinch of black pepper
- 2 chopped tomatoes
- 1 chopped onion
- Handful of chopped mint

How to make:

1. Pour the couscous into a bowl and add the cumin, smoked paprika and pinch of black pepper. Then grab a cup of boiling water and pour it over the couscous until it covers it by about 1cm. Cover the bowl and leave for around 10-15 minutes.
2. When the water has been absorbed, add the chopped chilli, chopped tomatoes, chopped mint and chopped onion to the bowl and stir.
3. Add the mackerel to the top and serve.

COD AND VEG

A simple recipe that's quick and easy to make and tasty too. You guessed it - high in protein and low in carbs!

Nutritional value

Calories per serving: 324
Protein: 28g
Carbs: 11g
Fat: 19g

Ingredients

- 140g fillet of white fish (boneless)
- Handful of frozen peas
- A pinch of salt and pepper
- 1 tbsp of olive oil
- 2 sliced spring onions
- 1 chopped gem lettuce
- 2 tbsp reduced-fat crème fraîche

How to make:

1. Add the lettuce, spring onions, frozen peas and olive oil to a microwave-proof bowl.
2. Season the fish with salt and pepper and 1 tbsp crème fraîche and add to the bowl.
3. Cover the bowl with cling film; pierce it several times with a fork and place in microwave.
4. Microwave the bowl for around 8 minutes until the fish as been fully cooked and is piping hot throughout.
5. Take the bowl from the microwave and remove the fish, placing to one side.
6. Use a fork to mash the vegetables and serve topped with the fish and an extra spoonful of crème fraîche.

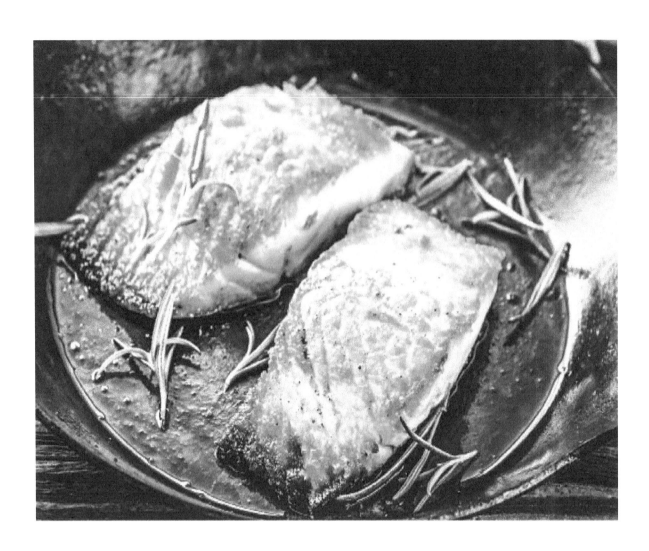

LEMONY SALMON

Salmon is a great source of protein and is very high in omega 3 fats. Most salmon dishes can be bland and boring...Not this one!

Nutritional value

(Serves 4)
Calories per serving: 205
Protein: 20g
Carbs: 1g
Fat: 13g

Ingredients

- 4 100g Salmon fillets
- 1 lemon
- A pinch of salt and pepper
- 10g of chopped tarragon
- Handful of rocket
- 2 tbsp of olive oil
- 1 chopped garlic clove

How to make:

1. Pre-Heat grill Get a bowl and add the chopped garlic, tarragon, sprinkle of salt, sprinkle of pepper and olive oil. Squeeze the lemon juice and zest in the bowl and mix everything together.
2. Add the salmon fillets to the bowl and coat them in the marinade. Cover the bowl and leave the salmon fillets to marinade for 10 minutes.
3. Take the salmon fillets out of the bowl and place on a tray, pouring the marinade over the top of the fillets.
4. Grill the salmon fillets for around 10 minutes or until cooked through.
5. Plate up and serve.

STRENGTHENING SUB-CONTINENTAL SARDINES

Sardines are a great source of protein as well as omega 3's.

Nutritional value

(Serves 4)
Calories per serving: 356
Protein: 20g
Carbs: 52g
Fat: 7g

Ingredients

- 50g plain flour
- 10 sardines, scaled and cleaned (8 if large)
- Zest of 2 whole lemons
- Handful of chopped flat-leaf parsley,
- 3 garlic cloves, finely chopped
- 3 tbsp olive oil
- 400g of tinned chopped tomatoes
- 800g chickpeas or butterbeans, drained and rinsed
- 250g pack cherry tomatoes, halved
- A pinch of salt and pepper

How to make:

1. Sprinkle the flour with salt and pepper and spread the flour out on the work surface.
2. Cover the sardines with the flour on each side.
3. Now in a separate bowl add the lemon zest to the chopped parsley (save a pinch for garnishing) and half of the chopped garlic, ready for later.
4. Put a very large pan on the grill and heat on high.
5. Now add the oil and once very hot, lay the floured sardines flat.
6. Fry for 3 minutes until golden underneath and turn over to fry for another 3 minutes. Put these onto a plate to rest.

7. Fry the remaining garlic (add another splash of oil if you need to) for 1 min until softened. Pour in the tin of chopped tomatoes, mix and let simmer for 4-5 minutes.
8. Tip in the chickpeas or butter beans and fresh tomatoes, then stir until heated through.
9. Here's when you add the sardines into the lemon and parsley mix and cook for a further 3-4 minutes.
10. Once they're cooked through, serve with a pinch of parsley to garnish.

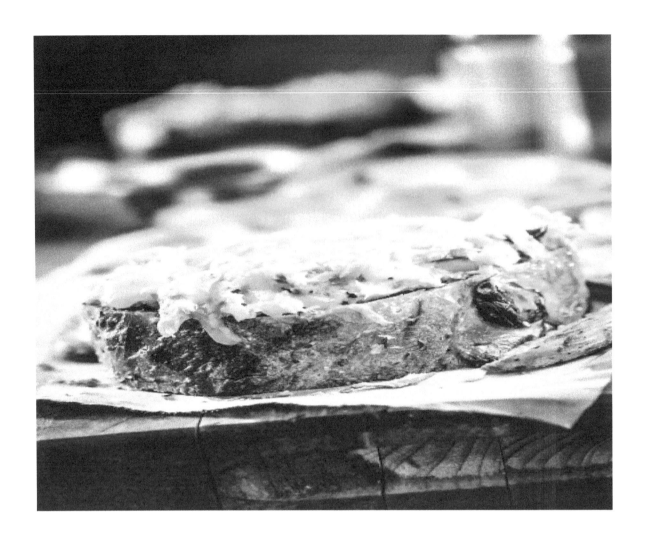

MIGHTY TUNA MELTS

Not sure what to do with that tuna can at the back of the cupboard? This is a delicious protein packed recipe that's ready in minutes.

Nutritional value

(Serves 2)
Calories per serving: 450
Protein: 37g
Carbs: 20g
Fat: 24g

Ingredients

• 200g of tinned, drained tuna
• 2 chopped spring onions stems
• 4 tbsp low-fat mayonnaise
• 4 thick slices Ezekial or wholemeal bread
• 50g grated low fat cheddar
• 2 tbsp of chilli flakes
• 1 squeezed lemon
• A pinch of salt and pepper

How to make:

1. Toast the bread and pre-heat the grill.
2. Get a bowl and add the spring onions, mayonnaise, tuna and chilli flakes along with salt and pepper and the lemon juice. Mix everything together.
3. Spread the tuna mix over the top of the slices of bread and sprinkle the grated cheese over the top. Place under the grill until the cheese starts to bubble.
4. Plate up and serve.

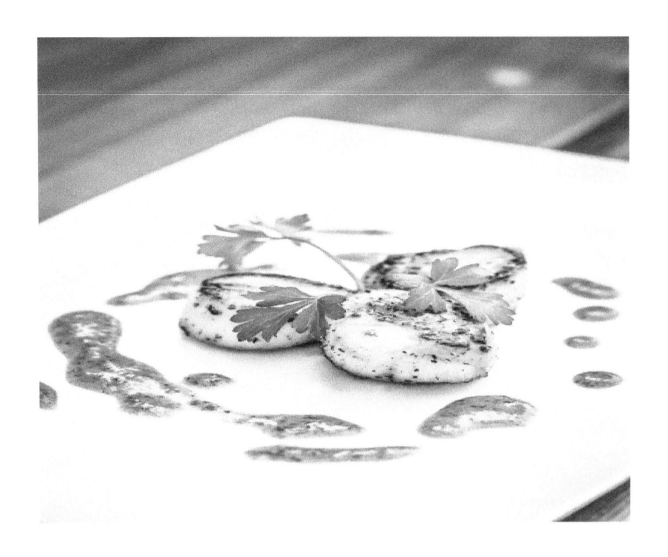

RUSTIC SCALLOPS WITH CORIANDER AND LIME

Scallops are a delicacy and if you feel like pushing the boat out, a great tasty change from the norm!

Nutritional value

Calories per serving: 225
Protein: 20g
Carbs: 3g
Fat: 14g

Ingredients

- 8 queen or king scallops (row on)
- 1 tbsp olive oil
- 2 large chopped garlic cloves
- 1 tsp chopped fresh red chilli
- 1/2 lime juice
- 2 tbsp of chopped coriander
- A pinch of salt and pepper

How to make:

1. Heat pan on a medium to high and fry scallops for about 1 minute each side until golden. Add the chopped chilli and garlic cloves to the pan and squeeze the lime juice over the scallops.
2. Remove the scallops and sprinkle the chilli and coriander over them as well as some salt and pepper to serve.

TRAINING TILAPIA IN THAI SAUCE

Tilapia is an exotic sounding fish but can often be found in your local fishmonger or superstore counter. Failing this, you can use this recipe with Sea Bass or any other fish fillets of your choice!

Nutritional value

(Serves 4)
Calories per serving: 328
Protein: 28g
Carbs: 25g
Fat: 14g

Ingredients

- 4 tilapia fillets
- 2 tbsp flour
- 2 tbsp olive oil
- 4 spring onion stems, sliced
- 1 stick of chopped lemon grass
- 2 crushed garlic cloves
- 1 thumb-size piece of chopped fresh ginger
- 2 tbsp soy sauce
- Lime juice of 1 lime, plus 1 lime chopped into wedges, to serve
- 1 chopped red chilli
- Handful of coriander leaves

How to make:

1. Dip the tilapia fillets into the flour so that the whole fillet is coated.
2. Add olive oil to a pan on a medium to high heat and fry the fillets for 3 minutes on each side.
3. Using the same pan, fry the garlic, chilli, lemon grass and ginger on a low heat, adding the soy sauce and lime juice and simmering until the sauce thickens slightly.
4. Spoon the sauce over the fish and add the spring onions for a couple

of minutes before dishing up and garnishing with your choice of herb and the lime wedges on the side.

TANGY TROUT

Trout is the king of all river fish and its goodness cannot be underrated! Sea trout is just as majestic so don't rule it out!

Nutritional value

Calories per serving: 298
Protein: 30g
Carbs: 10g
Fat: 16g

Ingredients

• 4 trout fillets
• 50g whole wheat/brown breadcrumbs (you can buy these pre-packaged or just use your trusty blender to wiz up your crust ends!)
• 1 tbsp olive oil
• 1 small chopped bunch parsley
• Zest and juice of 1 lemon
• 25g toasted and chopped pine nuts or walnuts

How to make:

1. Turn your grill up high.
2. In the meantime, spread a little oil over a baking tray and mix the breadcrumbs, parsley, lemon zest and juice and half of the nuts.
3. Lay the fillets skin side down onto your tray and rub into your mixture on both sides before drizzling with more olive oil.
4. Leave them under the grill for five minutes and then scatter over the rest of the nuts to serve.

STEAMY WORKOUT FISH

This dish is fresh and delicious; it's so easy to cook and you can pack it full with extra greens and vitamins!

Nutritional value

Serves 4
Calories per serving: 145
Protein: 29g
Carbs: 4g
Fat: 1g

Ingredients

• Tin foil, greaseproof paper or baking paper.
• 100g pak choi
• 4 x 150g fillets firm white fish (Cod, Plaice, Pollock, Seabass or Haddock)
• 2 garlic cloves, finely chopped
• 2 tbsp soy sauce
• 1 tsp mirin rice wine
• 4 chopped spring onions stems
• Handful of chopped coriander

How to make:

1. Heat oven to (200°C/400°F/Gas Mark 6).
2. You're going to be making a parcel for your delicious ingredients so you will need tin foil, greaseproof paper or baking paper.
3. Cut off four large rectangles and place each fillet on each piece of paper.
4. Add the garlic, soy sauce and rice wine.
5. You may want to use one or two of the lime wedges to squeeze the juices into your parcel.
6. Fold these up into a parcel leaving one edge open.
7. Cook for 20 minutes then add the spring onions and chilli for a fresh taste to end.

MUSCLE BUILDING SARDINES ON TOAST

A quick and easy muscle-building recipe to make: perfect for lunches or snacks.

Nutritional value

(Serves 2)
Calories per serving: 442
Protein: 24g
Carbs: 30g
Fat: 23g

Ingredients

• 4 slices Ezekiel bread or whole wheat brown bread
• 2 cans of drained sardines in olive oil
• 1 tbsp olive oil
• 1 chopped garlic clove
• 1 chopped red chilli
• 1 lemon, zest and juice
• Handful of chopped parsley

How to make:

1. Toast the bread.
2. Heat some olive oil in a pan on a medium heat.
3. Add the chilli, garlic, lemon zest and sardines and heat for 2-3 minutes until cooked.
4. Place the sardines on the toast and sprinkle the parsley over them. Finish off with a few drops of lemon juice to serve.

TASTY TUNA, BROCCOLI & CAULIFLOWER PASTA BAKE

Delicious pasta meal packed with protein for all your muscle-building and fat loss needs.

Nutritional value

(Serves 4)
Calories per serving: 641
Protein: 37g
Carbs: 73g
Fat: 22g

Ingredients

- 2 cans of tuna in olive oil (drained)
- 800g of canned chopped tomatoes
- 350g whole-wheat pasta
- 150g chopped broccoli
- 150g chopped cauliflower
- 200g pack light soft cheese
- 100g of grated cheddar
- 25g whole-wheat breadcrumbs
- 1 tbsp of olive oil

How to make:

1. Grab a pan and heat the olive oil (medium/high heat).
2. Add the canned tomatoes and 200ml of water and let simmer.
3. Heat another large pan of water until it boils. Add the whole-wheat pasta and leave until the pan starts to boil again. Reduce the heat until the water simmers. Leave the whole-wheat pasta to cook for around 10 minutes. Add the broccoli and cauliflower during the last 3 minutes then drain.
4. Whilst the pasta and veg is cooking, pre heat the grill.
5. Add the cheese to the tomato sauce and stir until it melts, then add the drained pasta, vegetables and tuna.

6. Pour the mixture in a deep tray and cover with the cheddar, breadcrumbs, salt and pepper.
7. Place under the grill and cook for 6 minutes until golden.
8. Plate up and serve.

BRAWNY BAKED HADDOCK WITH SPINACH AND PEA RISOTTO

Haddock is cheap and easy to cook and on top of this is packed full of nutrients and is a warm and wholesome filler!

Nutritional value

(Serves 4)
Calories per serving: 469
Protein: 32g
Carbs: 66g
Fat: 10g

Ingredients

• 400g skinless, boneless, smoked haddock from your local fishmonger or supermarket
• 1 tbsp olive oil
• 1 onion, chopped
• 300g risotto rice
• 450 ml of vegetable stock
• 250g fresh spinach leaves
• Handful of frozen peas
• 3 tbsp crème fraîche
• 50g grated parmesan cheese
• A pinch of pepper

How to make:

1. Heat the oil in a large pan or wok on a medium heat.
2. Fry the chopped onion until just soft (not brown) before adding in the rice and stirring until soft.
3. Now add half of the stock and continue to stir slowly until the rice takes on a translucent texture.
4. Keep adding the rest of the stock slowly whilst stirring for up to 20-30 minutes.

5. Stir in the spinach and peas to the risotto.
6. Place the fish on top of the rice, replace the lid, then let steam for 10 minutes.
7. Flake the fish into large chunks and stir into the rice with the crème fraîche and half the parmesan.
8. Sprinkle with freshly ground pepper, then add the rest of the parmesan on top to taste!

SUPER HUMAN SEA BASS WITH SIZZLING SPICES

A delicious meaty meal that's packed full of protein.

Nutritional value

(Serves 6)
Calories per serving: 202
Protein: 28g
Carbs: 2g
Fat: 9g

Ingredients

- 6 x sea bass fillets skin on and scaled
- 3 tbsp olive oil
- 1 thumb-size piece of ginger, peeled and chopped into slices
- 3 thinly sliced garlic cloves
- 3 red chillies deseeded and thinly sliced
- 5 sliced spring onion stems
- 1 tbsp soy sauce

How to make:

1. Get a large pan and heat 2 tbsp of the oil on a medium heat.
2. Sprinkle salt and pepper over the Sea Bass and score the skin of the fish a few times with a sharp knife.
3. Add the sea bass fillet to the very hot pan with the skin side down (you must press the fish down onto the pan with your cooking spatula to prevent the fish from shrivelling and shrinking).
4. Cook the fish this way for around 5 minutes, or until you can see the skin underneath turning golden brown (you can lose the pressure on the spatula after the first few seconds)!
5. Now turn the fish over for around 30 seconds to give the flesh a nice golden colour.
6. Take the fish out of the pan, and place to one side.
7. Add the rest of the oil to the pan, throw in the chillies, garlic and

ginger and cook for approximately 2 minutes or until golden.

8. Take this off the heat and add the spring onions with the soy sauce. Pour the sauce over your sea bass for a delicious oriental treat.

JOCK'S JACKET POTATO WITH TUNA

Who said a jacket potato had to be boring? Try this sweet potato version and you'll be left satisfied and full with your fair share of protein!

Nutritional value

Calories per serving: 352
Protein: 33g
Carbs: 27g
Fat: 13g

Ingredients

- 1 large sweet potato
- 185g can tuna in olive oil, drained
- ½ finely chopped red onion,
- 1 small deseeded and chopped red chilli, (dried chilli will be just as good)
- 1 tbsp natural yoghurt
- A bunch of chopped spring onions

How to make:

1. Preheat the oven to (200°C/400°F/Gas Mark 6).
2. You don't need to peel the sweet potato but you may want to scrape off the nobly bits with a sharp knife!
3. Pierce the potato with a fork multiple times and place in the microwave for 20 minutes (if you don't have a microwave you can use the oven but it will take around 30 minutes).
4. Whilst it's cooking, mix the tuna with the chopped onion and chill and season with salt and pepper.
5. Place the sweet potato in the pre-heated oven for a further 5-10 minutes or until a little crispy and serve with the tuna mix and yoghurt over the top.
6. Sprinkle the chopped spring onion over that!

CHAPTER 8: SALADS

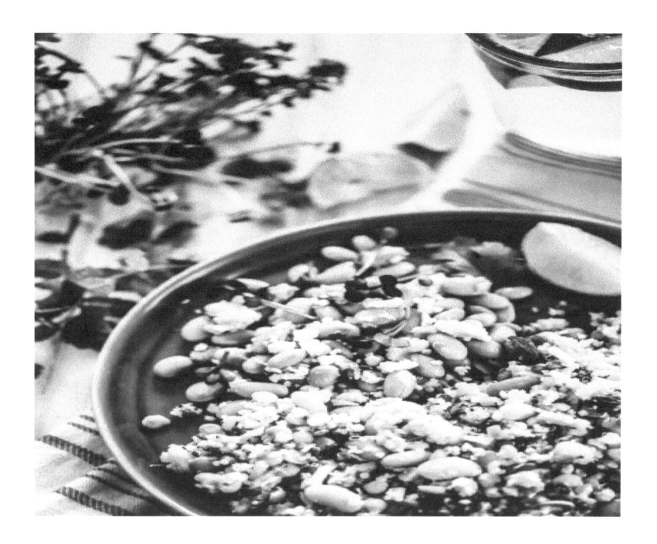

SALADS

Salads are boring right? They're only designed for rabbits and skinny women on diets. Wrong. Salads done right are firstly delicious and don't have to just be a side; secondly they can be stuffed with fibre, protein, vitamins, nutrients. Don't make the stupid error of ignoring our trusted training companions and try a salad soon.

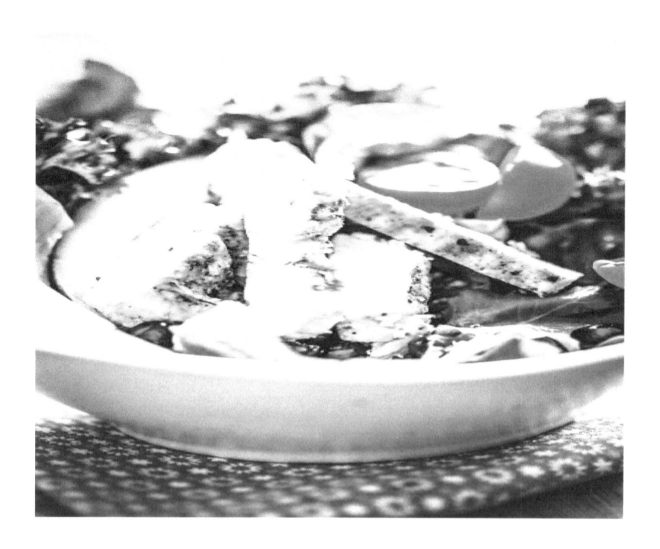

ANABOLIC AVOCADO AND CHICKEN SALAD

A fresh and delicious salad, pleasing the meat eater and keeping you anabolic!

Nutritional value

Calories per serving: 389
Protein: 36g
Carbs: 12g
Fat: 14g

Ingredients

- 1 chicken breast
- Handful of watercress
- Handful of baby spinach
- Handful of rocket
- ½ peeled and sliced avocado
- 1 chopped beef tomato
- ¼ sliced cucumber
- 2 tbsp of olive oil

How to make:

1. Heat some olive oil on a medium heat in a griddle pan.
2. Grill the chicken breast for about 10 minutes each side or until cooked through.
3. Cut the chicken breasts into chunks and serve with the watercress, spinach, rocket, tomato and sliced avocado.
4. Finish off the salad by drizzling over olive oil.

TUNA, SPINACH & QUINOA SALAD

Quick and easy, tasty tuna salad for your muscle building and fat loss needs.

Nutritional value

(Serves 2)
Calories per serving: 302
Protein: 18g
Carbs: 28g
Fat: 13g

Ingredients

- 2 cans of tinned tuna in olive oil
- Handful of baby spinach
- 1 chopped red onion
- 300g of chopped peppers
- 1 tbsp olive oil
- 1 chopped red chilli
- 225g of quinoa
- 350g of halved cherry tomatoes
- 20g of chopped black olives

How to make:

1. Add the quinoa to a large pan of boiling water and cook for 10 – 15 minutes until tender, then drain.
2. Heat oil in a pan on a medium heat and fry the onions, peppers and chilli until softened.
3. Get a bowl and add the drained quinoa, onion mix, tomatoes, tuna, baby spinach and olives and mix together.
4. Serve and enjoy

ROASTED BEETROOT, GOATS' CHEESE & EGG SALAD

Whether you love it or hate it, beetroot is a super food containing nutrients you rarely find in your five portions a day! Give it a go if you never have, or try this take on it if you're already a fan.

Nutritional value

Calories per serving: 363
Protein: 11g
Carbs: 18g
Fat: 28g

Ingredients

- 200g cooked chopped beetroot (not in vinegar)
- 2 tbsp olive oil
- Juice from 1 orange
- 2 eggs
- 1 tsp white wine vinegar
- 2 tbsp crème fraîche
- 1 tsp Dijon mustard
- A few stalks of dill, finely chopped (fresh or dried)
- 70g of baby gem lettuce
- Handful of walnuts
- 100g crumbled goats cheese
- A pinch of salt and pepper

How to make:

1. Preheat oven to (200°C/400°F/Gas Mark 6).
2. Place the beetroot onto the lightly oiled baking tray with the juice from the orange, sprinkle with salt and pepper.
3. Roast for 20-25 minutes, turning them once whilst they're baking. If they start to dry out, add a little more olive oil.
4. Meanwhile, put the eggs in boiling water. Turn down the heat and simmer for 8 minutes (4 minutes if you like your yolks runny) then

run under cold water to cool. Peel and halve.

5. Mix the remaining oil, crème fraîche, mustard, a tsp of white wine vinegar and chopped dill together. This is the dressing for your lettuce.

6. Serve the salad with the beetroot and goats cheese crumbled over the top and walnuts sprinkled throughout.

SPICY MEXICAN BEAN STEW

This one is technically a salad but really it could pass on anyone's dinner table. You won't be left hungry after this one and you'll certainly feel the heat kick-starting your metabolism!

Nutritional value

(Serves 4)
Calories per serving: 395
Protein: 20g
Carbs: 45g
Fat: 15g

Ingredients

- 250g canned chick peas, drained
- 200g canned cannellini beans, drained
- 200g of tinned chopped tomatoes
- 2 tbsp olive oil
- 1 chopped red onion
- 190g of sliced chorizo
- 3 red chopped chillis
- 1 tbsp paprika

How to make:

1. Heat a large pan on a medium heat with 1 tbsp olive oil, and cook the onion and chorizo for 5 minutes until lightly golden.
2. Tip in the chickpeas with the cannellini beans and stir until heated through.
3. Add the tin of chopped tomatoes and paprika and cover to let simmer for 5-10 minutes.
4. Serve – recommended with crusty brown bread, couscous or brown rice for a winter warmer!

THE SAILOR SALAD

Spinach was good enough for the well-known muscle-building sailor cartoon then and its more than good enough for you now; add a generous portion of the sailor's catch and you'll be growing bigger than he ever did.

Nutritional value

(Serves 4)
Calories per serving: 220
Protein: 20g
Carbs: 12.5g
Fat: 10g

Ingredients

• 100g of chopped spinach (fresh)
• 170g of lean grilled chopped turkey breast (or turkey deli meat already cooked)
• 1 tbsp real bacon bits (you can cut up bacon and grill this yourself or buy the pre-packaged stuff)
• 2 diced hard-boiled eggs
• 100g baby potatoes
• 1 deseeded and sliced red, yellow and green pepper
• 1 avocado peeled and sliced (do this near to the end or it will start to turn brown)
• 1 tbsp balsamic vinegar
• A pinch of salt and pepper

How to make:

1. Boil a medium sized pan of water on a high heat and add the halved new potatoes, cooking for 15-20 minutes or according to packaging guidelines.
2. Combine the meats (once grilled and chopped if you're doing this yourself) with the spinach and peppers in a serving bowl.
3. Drain the potatoes and let cool whilst placing a small pan to boil for

the eggs. Cook for 8 minutes for medium-boiled or 10 minutes for hard-boiled eggs.

4. Run the eggs under a cold tap and peel. Dice and add to your salad (here's where you can peel the avocado and add this).

5. Stir through with balsamic vinegar and salt and pepper to taste.

SIZZLING SALMON SALAD

*Some like it hot. You can serve this one up with warm or cold salmon –
either way it's wholesome and mouth-watering.*

Nutritional value

Calories per serving: 521
Protein: 46g
Carbs: 24g
Fat: 27g

Ingredients

• 150g fillet salmon
• 6 cherry tomatoes
• 100g of couscous
• 3 stems of asparagus (chop off the very end of the base but leave the rest intact)
• 50g of diced low-fat mozzarella cheese
• 1 bell pepper sliced
• 1 tbsp balsamic vinegar
• 1 tbsp olive oil
• A pinch of salt and pepper

How to make:

1. Preheat the grill.
2. Layer the couscous with boiling water from the kettle (about 1cm over the top of the couscous, cover and leave to steam)
3. Grill salmon for 10-15 minutes or until cooked through. Place to one side.
4. Uncover the couscous and stir through with a fork to break up the grains.
5. Now just add your pepper, mozzarella and halved cherry tomatoes to the couscous.
6. You will need to grill your asparagus for 3-4 minutes, turning every

so often until lightly browned around the surface.

7. Once the asparagus is ready, place it along with the salmon on the bed of couscous and drizzle with olive oil and balsamic vinegar.

8. Salt and pepper to taste.

HERBY TUNA STEAK

Protein, protein, protein!

Nutritional value

(Serves 2)
Calories per serving: 578
Protein: 35g
Carbs: 3g
Fat: 48g

Ingredients

- 2x 200g dolphin-friendly yellow fin tuna steaks
- 1 tbsp olive oil
- 2 lemon wedges
- 2 handfuls of flat-leaf parsley and 2 handfuls of coriander very roughly chopped
- 2 cloves of finely chopped garlic
- ½ onion finely chopped
- Handful chopped green olives
- 6 tbsp olive oil
- 50g pine nuts or walnuts
- Juice of half a lemon

How to make:

1. Your first job is the herby salad – mix the herbs with half of the chopped garlic, lemon juice and olive oil.
2. Crush the nuts in a tea towel or blend them up in your blender. Stir them in to the herbs.
3. Brush the tuna steaks with olive oil and sprinkle with salt and pepper.
4. You need to heat dry pan to an extremely high heat (look out for the smoke)
5. Seal the tuna in the pan for one minute on each side (if you have a

griddle pan or grill then you should place these against the lines to get that nice straight off the BBQ look and taste)

6. If you like your tuna less-pink cook for 2 minutes on each side for medium, 3 for medium well and 4 for well done (approximate times).

7. Once cooked serve straight away with your herby salad (pour this over as a dressing or on the side as an accompaniment)

MEDITERRANEAN SUPER SALAD

Quinoa's goodness cannot be overstated, this salad is packed full of protein and is also delicious too!

Nutritional value

Calories per serving: 290
Protein: 15g
Carbs: 35g
Fat: 10g

Ingredients

• 200g quinoa
• 1 tsp olive oil
• ½ red onion, finely chopped
• 2 tbsp mint (fresh or dried) and roughly chopped
• 400g of Puy or Red lentils rinsed and drained – you can buy the dried lentils but you need to leave them to soak over night.
• ¼ cucumber (skin off and diced)
• 100g crumbled feta cheese
• Zest and juice of 1 orange
• 1 tbsp red or white wine vinegar

How to make:

1. Cook the quinoa in a large pan of boiling water for 10-15 minutes until soft, drain and set aside to cool.
2. Fry the onion in the oil over a medium heat.
3. Stir together with the quinoa, lentils, cucumber, feta, orange zest, chopped mint and juice and vinegar.
4. Best served chilled!
5. For the meat fans, cooked chicken or lamb would be a delicious addition to this dish!

MUSCLE BUILDING STEAK & CHEESE SALAD

A very quick and easy, healthy muscle building salad.

Nutritional value

(Serves 2)
Calories per serving: 308
Protein: 34g
Carbs: 15g
Fat: 14g

Ingredients

- 250 frying beef steak
- 1 chopped red onion
- 1 teaspoon of crushed garlic
- Handful of baby spinach
- Handful of watercress
- Handful of lettuce
- 4 chopped baby tomatoes
- 2 tbsp of balsamic vinegar
- 1 tbsp olive oil
- 50g of blue cheese
- A pinch of salt and pepper

How to make:

1. Sprinkle salt and pepper over the steak.
2. Add a tbsp of olive oil to a griddle pan on a high heat.
3. Place the steak in the pan and cook 8 minutes in total, turning the steak half way through. Take the steak off the pan and allow to cool.
4. Cut the steak into 2cm strips, then place back into the pan and cook for a further minute on a medium heat.
5. Get a bowl and add the chopped tomatoes, watercress, baby spinach, lettuce, garlic and onions. Place the steak strips in the bowl along with the vinegar and a tbsp of olive oil. Mix everything together and

grate the blue cheese over the top.

HUNKED UP HALLOUMI

This cheese could almost be meat it's so chunky and filling!

Nutritional value

(Serves 4)
Calories per serving: 461
Protein: 29g
Carbs: 3g
Fat: 37g

Ingredients

- 2 tbsp white wine vinegar
- 2 tsp olive oil
- ½ red onion thinly sliced
- Handful of rocket leaves
- ½ juiced lemon
- Handful of green/black olives
- 500g of sliced halloumi cheese
- 1 tbsp mayonnaise
- ½ chopped cucumber
- A pinch of pepper

How to make:

1. Preheat the grill.
2. Lightly drizzle a baking tray with 1 tsp olive oil before grilling for 5 minutes, turning until browned and crisp on the edges.
3. Add the chopped olives, rocket, cucumber and red onion into a bowl and mix with 1 tsp olive oil and lemon juice.
4. Season with pepper and stir in the mayonnaise (optional).
5. Serve alone or with crusty brown pitta breads for an Aegean twist!

STRENGTH CHICKEN AND SESAME SALAD

Contains three sources of protein for all your muscle-building needs.

Nutritional value

(Serves 2)
Calories per serving: 430
Protein: 20g
Carbs: 16g
Fat: 15g

Ingredients

- 2 chicken breasts
- 3 tbsp of sesame oil
- 2 tsp of grated ginger
- 1 crushed garlic clove
- 1 chopped red chilli
- 1 diced red onion
- Handful of basil leaves
- Handful of coriander leaves
- 100g of baby spinach leaves
- 1 tsp of sesame seeds
- 4 chopped almonds
- 1 peeled and sliced mandarin

How to make:

1. Pre-heat the grill.
2. Add 2 tbsp sesame oil, chopped red chilli, crushed garlic and ginger into a bowl. Mix all the ingredients together.
3. Make a few deep cuts into the chicken breast and leave them to marinate in the mixture for roughly 3 hours.
4. Add the spinach leaves, coriander leaves, basil leaves, red onion, chopped almonds and sesame seeds to a bowl and mix together.
5. Remove the chicken and rub over the last of the marinade and grill

for 10 minutes each side or until fully cooked.

6. Cut the chicken into strips and add to the salad bowl.

7. Add the mandarin to the bowl and drizzle 1 tbsp of sesame oil over the salad and serve.

CHAPTER 9: SIDES

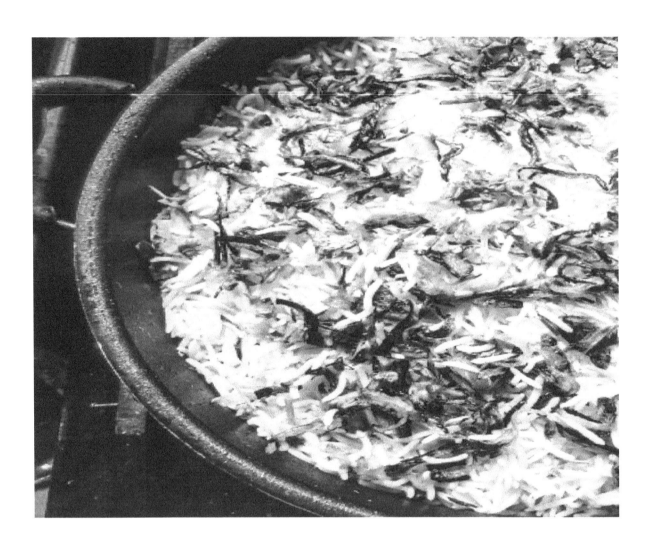

SIDES

Not enough to fill you up? Craving your side order of fries? Eyes bigger than your belly? No sweat. Here's a sweet collection of side orders you can prepare in your own home – add calories, protein and a little extra something, whilst knowing you've made it in the healthy way.

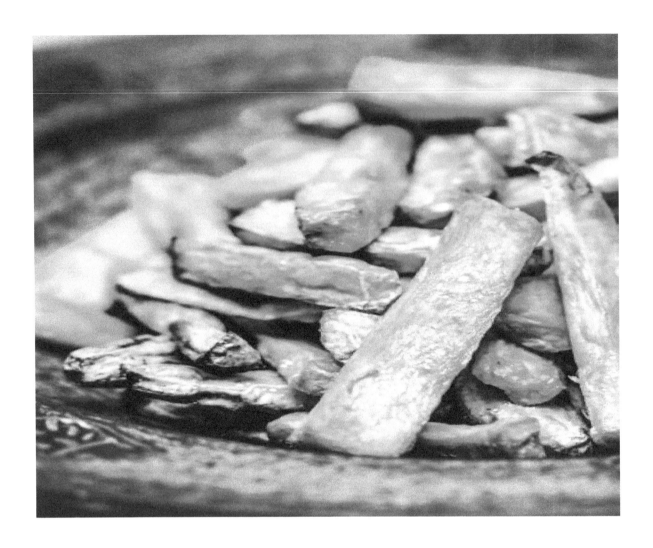

SWEET POTATO WEDGES

You won't be the only one devouring these tasty wedges.

Nutritional value

Calories per serving: 207
Protein: 3g
Carbs: 38g
Fat: 6g

Ingredients

• 4 sweet potatoes, scrubbed and cut into large wedges
• 2 tbsp olive oil
• 3-4 cloves of garlic
• Handful of rosemary sprigs

How to make:

1. Pre-heat oven to (350°F/180 °C/Gas Mark 4).
2. Once you've scrubbed the skin of the sweet potatoes (don't remove it) with a kitchen scourer or something rough to suffice, you should toss the wedges in olive oil.
3. Spread these out on a baking tray, sprinkling the rosemary sprigs over the wedges and adding the whole garlic cloves in their skin over and around the wedges. Pop the whole lot into a pre-heated oven for 30-40 minutes or until crispy.

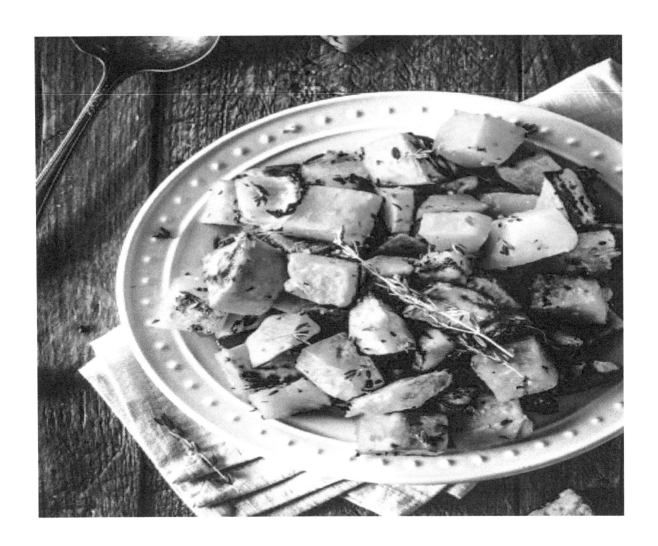

HOT & SPICY BUTTERNUT SQUASH

Often ignored in our fruit and veg selection, squash is a winner! One squash will feed a family, and if you're dining solo, freeze and save for another day!

Nutritional value

(Serves 4)
Calories per serving: 227
Protein: 1g
Carbs: 30g
Fat: 14g

Ingredients

- 1 butternut squash
- 4 tbsp olive oil
- 4 tbsp pouring honey
- 1 deseeded and finely chopped red scotch bonnet chilli

How to make:

1. Preheat the oven to (200°C/400°F/gas 6).
2. Chop the top and the bottom from the butternut squash. Next you need to cut it in half lengthways. You should now be able to use a vegetable peeler to remove the skin but if that doesn't work, take a sharp knife and cut downwards.
3. Now, using a spoon hollow out the seeds from the base.
4. You're free to slice now into thick (1-2 cm) slices horizontally.
5. On a lightly oiled baking tray, spread the slices into one layer across.
6. Drizzle the honey generously over the slices and sprinkle the chopped chili liberally (or according to heat tolerance!)
7. Bake for 35-40 minutes or until crispy.
8. Any left overs can be placed into a sealable sandwich bag and frozen – simply reheat in the oven when ready.

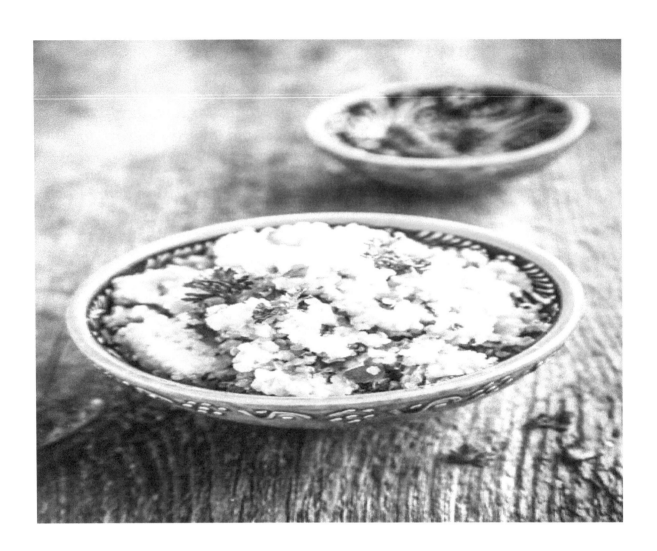

FRUITY NUTTY QUINOA

Don't know what to do with your quinoa? This dish is absolutely delicious and will go great with most main meals

Nutritional value

(Serves 4)
Calories per serving: 328
Protein: 10g
Carbs: 36g
Fat: 15g

Ingredients

- 200g quinoa
- 6 dried apricots
- Juice of 1 lemon
- 2 tbsp olive oil
- A pinch of salt and pepper
- Handful of chopped parsley and mint
- 50g cashew nuts

How to make:

1. Add the quinoa to a large pan of boiling water and then let simmer for 10 – 15 minutes until tender, then drain.
2. Get a bowl and add the quinoa, apricots, herbs, lemon juice, zest and olive oil along with some salt and pepper and mix together.
3. Scatter the cashews over the top and serve.

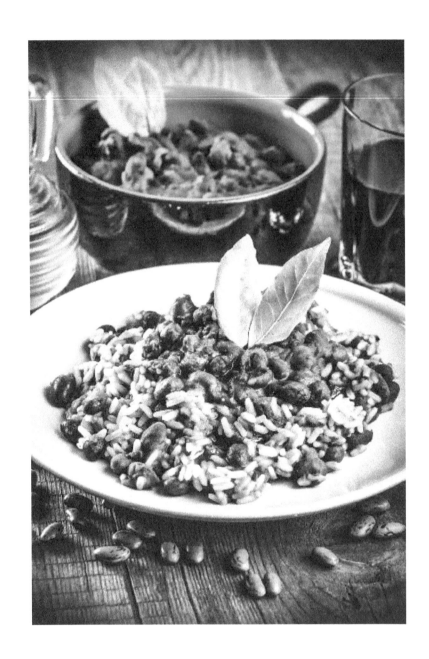

RICE & PEAS

Transport yourself to the Caribbean with this easy to prepare side dish.

Nutritional value

(Serves 2)
Calories per serving: 430
Protein: 20g
Carbs: 16g
Fat: 15g

Ingredients

- 300g brown rice
- 75ml olive oil
- 200g dried kidney beans
- 1 tsp chilli powder

How to make:

1. Soak the kidney beans in water overnight (you can buy tinned and use immediately if you're in a rush but you won't get that authentic color or taste!)
2. Boil the liquid with the kidney beans in using a large saucepan on a high heat (add water if you need to).
3. Add the rice and cook for 30 minutes and then drain. Keep the rice in the pan, add the kidney beans and cover and steam for 4 minutes.
4. Sprinkle chilli powder over your rice and serve

MUSCLE RICE SALAD

Add variety to your standard brown rice with this delicious and nutritious side.

Nutritional value

(Serves 2)
Calories per serving: 454
Protein: 11g
Carbs: 64g
Fat: 19g

Ingredients

- 100g of brown rice
- 1 deseeded and finely chopped red pepper,
- ½ cucumber finely chopped
- 1 large grated carrot
- 10 chopped cherry tomatoes
- 2 tbsp olive oil

How to make:

1. Add 300ml of cold water to a pot and heat on high until the water is boiling.
2. Once boiling, add the rice and leave for 20 minutes. Then drain.
3. Mix the rice with chopped red pepper, chopped cucumber, grated carrot, cherry tomatoes and drizzle with olive oil.

LEMON AND MOROCCAN MINT COUSCOUS

A fresh and zingy side dish that works well with fish, chicken, vegetables, and even lamb and beef.

Nutritional value

(Serves 2)
Calories per serving: 367
Protein: 6g
Carbs: 43g
Fat: 20g

Ingredients

• 250g couscous
• 2 tbsp grated zest of a lemon and the lemon juice
• 20g fresh mint
• 4 tbsp toasted pine nuts

How to make:

1. In a serving bowl, pour boiling water over the dried couscous (it needs to cover the couscous with about a cm on the top) and cover the bowl with a plate to steam. You could add a chicken/vegetable stock cube to the boiling water for seasoning if you wish.
2. Once the couscous has steamed for a few minutes uncover it and use a fork to 'fluff up' the grains.
3. Add the lemon zest and juice, finely chopped mint and pine nuts.
4. Season to taste and add a little olive oil to serve.

MUSHROOM RISOTTO

Another dish that works well on the side – try it with chicken breast. Works great as a post workout side!

Nutritional value

(Serves 2)
Calories per serving: 445
Protein: 15g
Carbs: 63g
Fat: 17g

Ingredients

• 50g dried porcini mushrooms
• 250g sliced and washed pack chestnut mushrooms
• 2 tbsp olive oil
• 1 finely chopped onion,
• 2 finely chopped garlic cloves,
• 300g risotto rice, such as Arborio
• 175ml white wine
• Handful tarragon leaves chopped
• 50g freshly grated parmesan or grana padano,

How to make:

1. Pour 1 litre of boiling water over the dried porcini mushrooms and leave to soak for 20 minutes, then drain into a separate bowl (keep the liquid at this point as you need to add to the risotto later).
2. Chop the mushrooms into slices.
3. Heat up the oil on a medium heat in a large frying pan and add the onions and garlic, frying for around 5 minutes until they get soft.
4. At this point you should add the dried and fresh chestnut mushrooms and stir for another 5 minutes until softened.
5. Add the rice, stirring for a minute or so before adding all of the wine.

6. Let it get to simmering point (bubbling), and add a quarter of the mushroom stock.
7. Simmer the rice, stirring often, until the rice has absorbed all the liquid.
8. Keep adding the stock, a quarter at a time, each time waiting for the rice to absorb the liquid.
9. A lot of stirring is required until the rice is soft! If the liquid runs out and the rice is still a little hard you can continue to add small amounts of water.
10. When soft, take the pan off the heat and add half the cheese and tarragon leaves. Cover the pan and let it steam for a few minutes.
11. Serve with the rest of the cheese and herbs!

SWEDE AND CARROT MASH UP

Try this home comfort – it's exciting mash!

Nutritional value

(Serves 4)
Calories per serving: 132
Protein: 2g
Carbs: 22g
Fat: 5g

Ingredients

- 500g chopped carrots
- 500g chopped swede
- 3 chopped garlic cloves
- Handful of finely chopped tarragon,
- 1 tbsp. olive oil
- A pinch of salt and pepper

How to make:

1. MUSTARDY CAULIFLOWER CHEESE
2. A Winter Warmer – eat alone or on the side.
3. Nutritional value
4. (Serves 2)
5. Calories per serving: 240

Protein: 15g
Carbs: 14g
Fat: 12g
Ingredients
- 1 whole cauliflower
- 2 tbsp wholegrain mustard
- 100g low fat cheddar cheese
- 100ml low-fat crème fraiche
How to make:

- Chop the cauliflower by cutting off the thickest part of the stem and pulling apart the florets.
- In a mixing bowl, place the cauliflower, ¾ of the cheese, crème fraîche and mustard and toss.
- Place in an oven dish and pop into a preheated oven (200°C/400°F/gas 6) for 30 minutes.
- Add the remaining cheese on to the top of the dish and grill for 5-7 minutes until brown and bubbling on top.

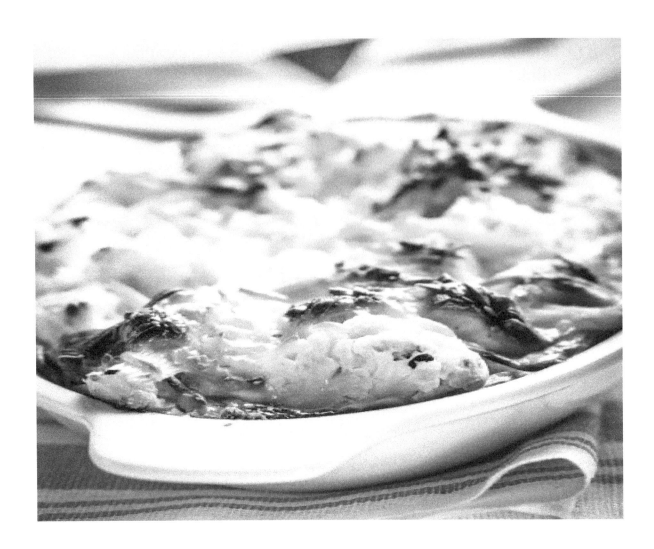

MUSTARDY CAULIFLOWER CHEESE

A Winter Warmer – eat alone or on the side.

Nutritional value

(Serves 2)
Calories per serving: 240
Protein: 15g
Carbs: 14g
Fat: 12g

Ingredients

- 1 whole cauliflower
- 2 tbsp wholegrain mustard
- 100g low fat cheddar cheese
- 100ml low-fat crème fraiche

How to make:

1. Chop the cauliflower by cutting off the thickest part of the stem and pulling apart the florets.
2. In a mixing bowl, place the cauliflower, ¾ of the cheese, crème fraîche and mustard and toss.
3. Place in an oven dish and pop into a preheated oven (200°C/400°F/gas 6) for 30 minutes.
4. Add the remaining cheese on to the top of the dish and grill for 5-7 minutes until brown and bubbling on top.

CHAPTER 10: HOMEMADE PROTEIN SHAKES

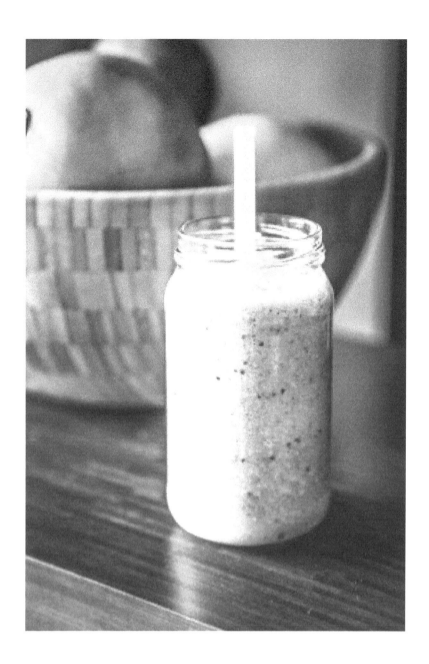

HOMEMADE PROTEIN SHAKES

If you want to spend hundreds of pounds on pre-made shakes full of chemicals and fillers that cements onto your kitchen sink then be my guest! If not, try these homemade healthy alternatives that will pack on just as much punch as the shop-bought varieties.

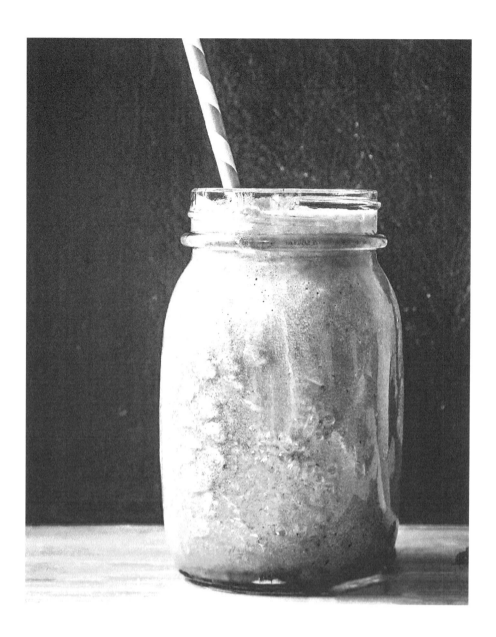

JASON'S HOMEMADE MASS GAINER

It can be hard to get all of the necessary calories to grow. Most weight-gainers contain empty calories and can be expensive. This beast of a shake contains around 1000 healthy calories and a whopping 75g of Protein to keep you growing.

Nutritional value

Calories per serving: 970
Protein:75g
Carbs: 90g
Fat: 30g

Ingredients

• 2 scoop of chocolate whey protein powder
• 2 cups of whole milk
• ½ cup of dry rolled oats
• 1 whole banana
• 2 tbsp of organic almond butter
• 1 cup of crushed ice

How to make:

1. Add all the ingredients to a blender and blend until smooth.
2. Enjoy.

CHOCOLATE PEANUT DELIGHT

Get your chocolate fix with this tasty shake.

Nutritional value

Calories per serving: 656
Protein: 63g
Carbs: 55g
Fat: 21g

Ingredients

- 1 scoop of chocolate whey protein powder
- 1 cup of low-fat Greek yogurt
- 1 whole banana
- 2 tbsp of peanut butter
- 1 cup of ice

How to make:

1. Add all the ingredients to a blender and blend until smooth.
2. Enjoy.

BERRY PROTEIN SHAKE

Totally refreshing on a hot summer's day and it works well any time of the year.

Nutritional value

Calories per serving: 342
Protein: 38g
Carbs: 42g
Fat: 3g

Ingredients

- 2 scoop of whey protein powder
- 1 cup of blueberries
- 1 cup of blackberries
- 1 cup of raspberries
- 1 cup of water
- 1 cup of ice

How to make:

1. Add all the ingredients to a blender and blend until smooth.
2. Enjoy.

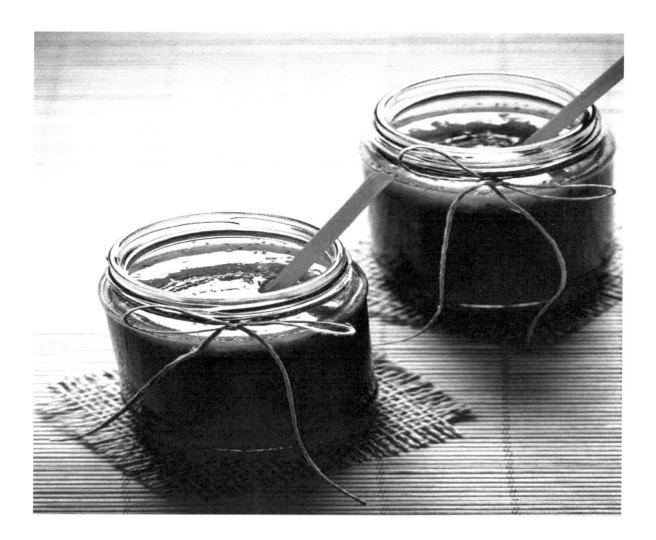

FRESH STRAWBERRY SHAKE

Keep it simple with this strawberry shake all year round.

Nutritional value

Calories per serving: 303
Protein: 35g
Carbs: 15g
Fat: 11g

Ingredients

• 2 scoops of vanilla protein powder
• 1 cup of strawberries
• 2 cups of water
• 1 tbsp of flaxseed oil

How to make:

1. Add all the ingredients to a blender and blend until smooth.
2. Enjoy.

CHOCO COFFEE ENERGY SHAKE

Swap your average morning caffeine hit with this refreshing alternative.

Nutritional value

Calories per serving: 299
Protein: 42g
Carbs: 14g
Fat: 6g

Ingredients

• 2 scoops of chocolate protein powder
• 100ml of low-fat milk
• 1 cup of water
• 1 tbsp of instant coffee

How to make:

1. Add all the ingredients to a blender and blend until smooth.
2. Enjoy.

LEAN AND MEAN PINEAPPLE SHAKE

Fresh, tropical and zingy – this shake really packs a punch and is crammed full of energy to keep you going until at least lunch!

Nutritional value

Calories per serving: 355
Protein: 23g
Carbs: 65g
Fat: 3g

Ingredients

- 1 cup chopped pineapple
- 4 strawberries
- 1 banana
- 1 tbsp low-fat Greek yogurt
- 1 scoop of vanilla protein powder
- 1 cup of water

How to make:

1. Add all the ingredients to a blender and blend until smooth.
2. Enjoy.

CHOPPED ALMOND SMOOTHIE

A quick and easy shake that will ease your chocolate craving and provide you with 24 grams of protein.

Nutritional value

Calories per serving: 241
Protein: 24g
Carbs: 6g
Fat: 13g

Ingredients

- 1 ½ cups water
- 17 chopped almonds
- ½ tsp coconut extract
- 1 scoop chocolate protein powder

How to make:

1. Add all the ingredients to a blender and blend until smooth.
2. Enjoy.

VANILLA STRAWBERRY SURPRISE

If this doesn't transport you back to a day out by the seaside nothing will – it tastes amazing and is deceptively good at filling you up and helping you to bulk up and shred fat.

Nutritional value

Calories per serving: 329
Protein: 36g
Carbs: 42g
Fat: 2g

Ingredients

- 2 scoops of vanilla protein powder
- 1 cup of ice
- 1 banana
- 4 fresh or frozen strawberries

How to make:

1. Add all the ingredients to a blender and blend until smooth.
2. Enjoy.

BREAKFAST BANANA SHAKE

Not much time? This breakfast shake packs a punch and will ensure a positive start to your day

Nutritional value

Calories per serving: 566
Protein: 59g
Carbs: 69g
Fat: 6g

Ingredients

- 200ml low-fat milk
- 1 banana
- 100g of rolled oats
- 2 scoops of vanilla whey protein powder

How to make:

1. Add all the ingredients to a blender and blend until smooth.
2. Enjoy.

PEACHY PUNCH

This peachy punch will satisfy your sweet tooth as well as providing 50 grams of protein.

Nutritional value

Calories per serving: 543
Protein: 50g
Carbs: 57g
Fat: 11g

Ingredients

- 2 scoop of vanilla protein powder
- 200ml of low-fat milk
- 45g of rolled oats
- 1 chopped peach
- 1 cup of water
- 50g of low fat Greek yogurt

How to make:

1. Add all the ingredients to a blender and blend until smooth.
2. Enjoy.

BLACKBERRY BRAWN

Quick and easy shake that is as tasty as it is nutritious.

Nutritional value

Calories per serving: 457
Protein: 47g
Carbs: 30g
Fat: 16g

Ingredients

- 1 cup of blackberries
- 200ml of low–fat milk
- 2 tbsp of Flax Seed oil
- 50g of low-fat Greek yogurt
- 2 scoops of vanilla protein powder
- 1 cup ice

How to make:

1. Add all the ingredients to a blender and blend until smooth.
2. Enjoy.

NO WHEY!

No protein powder? This healthy, tasty shake contains a dose of protein to keep you growing!

Nutritional value

Calories per serving: 388
Protein: 26g
Carbs: 32g
Fat: 22g

Ingredients

- 1 cup of blackberries
- 1 cup of strawberries
- 200ml of low–fat milk
- 130g of Greek yogurt
- 1 tbsp of almond butter
- 1 cup Ice

How to make:

1. Add all the ingredients to a blender and blend until smooth.
2. Enjoy.

CARIBBEAN CRUSH

Absolutely delicious!

Nutritional value

Calories per serving: 263
Protein: 25g
Carbs: 38g
Fat: 3g

Ingredients

- 1 scoop of protein powder (your choice)
- ½ chopped mango
- ½ cup of pineapple chunks
- 1 peeled and cubed kiwi
- 1 strawberry
- 1 cup of ice

How to make:

1. Add all the ingredients to a blender and blend until smooth.
2. Enjoy.

CHOCOLATE & RASPBERRY BANG

A tasty, quick protein shake to keep you growing and shredding!

Nutritional value

Calories per serving: 269
Protein: 31g
Carbs: 16g
Fat: 9g

Ingredients

• 2 scoops of chocolate protein powder
• ½ cup of raspberries
• 200ml of whole milk
• ½ cup of ice cubes

How to make:

1. Add all the ingredients to a blender and blend until smooth.
2. Enjoy.

CINNAMON SURPRISE

Quick and easy protein shake to satisfy your taste buds!

Nutritional value

Calories per serving: 244
Protein: 47g
Carbs: 7g
Fat: 4g

Ingredients

• 2 scoops of chocolate protein powder
• 1 tbsp of cinnamon
• 1 cup of water
• 1 cup of ice

How to make:

1. Add all the ingredients to a blender and blend until smooth.
2. Enjoy.

PUMPKIN POWER

A great tasting shake that's packed full of protein.

Nutritional value

Calories per serving: 224
Protein: 38g
Carbs: 14g
Fat: 3g

Ingredients

- 2 scoops of vanilla protein powder
- 1 cup of chopped pumpkin
- 1 tsp cinnamon
- 1 cup of water

How to make:

1. Add all the ingredients to a blender and blend until smooth.
2. Enjoy.

CHAPTER 11: DESSERTS

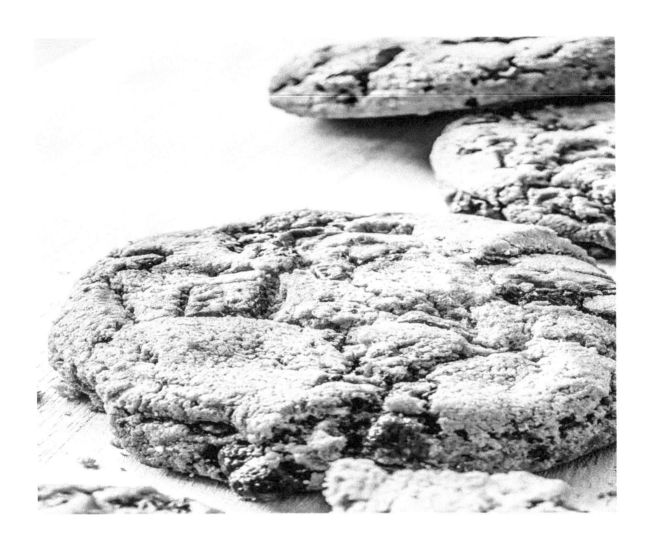

DESSERTS

Just because you are trying to build muscles doesn't mean you cannot indulge in sweet goodies once in a while. There are vegetarian desserts that are not only healthy, but rich in protein as well. Thus, your fitness goals will not be compromised. Here are some dessert recipes that you can try.

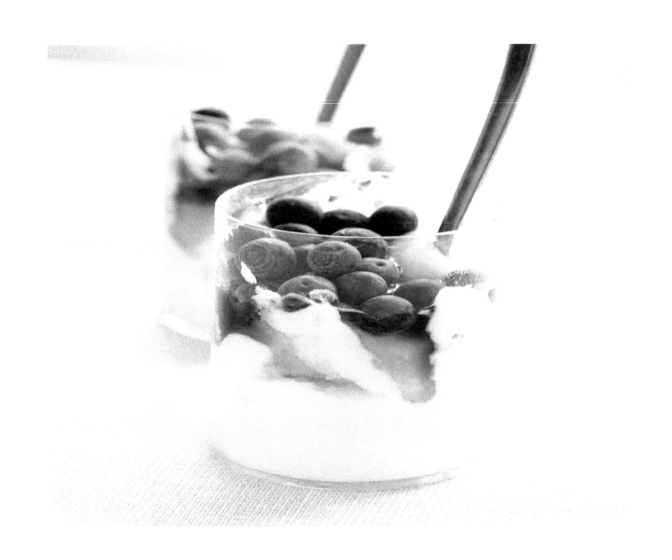

POWER PARFAIT

A delicious dessert that tastes a great as it looks. Contains a whopping 38g of protein.

Nutritional value

Calories per serving: 254
Protein: 38g
Carbs: 21g
Fat: 2g

Ingredients

• 1 scoop of vanilla protein powder
• 50g of mixed berries
• 200ml of Greek yogurt

How to make:

1. Mix the yogurt with the protein powder.
2. Get a tall parfait glass and layer with berries and yogurt.

GREEK YOGURT WITH HONEY AND BERRIES

A quick and easy dessert that contains a whopping 43g of protein. .

Nutritional value

Calories per serving: 522
Protein: 43g
Carbs: 86g
Fat: 7g

Ingredients

- 1 scoop of vanilla protein powder
- 100g Greek Yoghurt
- 4 tbsp of honey
- 45g of berries

How to make:

1. Mix all your ingredients and you've got a fresh and healthy dessert with nothing on your conscience. You could sprinkle flaked almonds over the top for a bit of crunch.

COTTAGE CHEESECAKE

A hearty, protein packed cheesecake to enjoy!

Nutritional value

Calories per serving: 487
Protein: 43g
Carbs: 53g
Fat: 7g

Ingredients

- 150g of fat free cottage cheese
- 1 scoop of vanilla protein powder
- 1 packet of stevia
- 1 tbsp sugar free instant pudding mix
- 5 tbsp of low fat milk
- Handful of Strawberries

How to make:

1. Add all the ingredients to a blender and blend until smooth.
2. Place in a bowl and top with the strawberries.

JASON'S PEANUT PROTEIN BARS

Save your money with these delicious, homemade protein bars!

Nutritional value

(Makes 12 bars)
Calories per bar: 386
Protein: 18g
Carbs: 24g
Fat: 6g

Ingredients

- 4 scoops of vanilla protein powder
- 400g of rolled oats
- 340g of almond butter
- 250ml of coconut cream

How to make:

1. Get a bowl and add the coconut cream and whisk until smooth, then add the protein powder and almond butter and mix thoroughly.
2. Pour the oats into the bowl and again mix thorough.
3. Scoop out the mixture into a baking tray and flatten until the surface is smooth
4. Place the tray in the fridge and leave for around 8 hours.
5. Cut into 12 bars.

BANANA PROTEIN PUDDING

I would recommend this all the time, but if you want to treat yourself, this is a quick and easy pudding that tastes great and contains a healthy dose of protein.

Nutritional value

(Serves 4)
Calories per serving: 357
Protein: 30g
Carbs: 22g
Fat: 20g

Ingredients

• 100g low-fat butter
• 4 scoops of vanilla protein powder
• 2 chopped bananas
• 100g self-raising flour
• 2 tsp ground cinnamon
• 2 eggs
• 2 tbsp low fat milk

How to make:

1. Get a dish and scoop in the butter. Place in the microwave for 30 seconds until melted. Mash 1 banana in the bowl. Then add the protein powder, flour, cinnamon, eggs, milk and mix together.
2. Place the other chopped banana over the top of the mix. Place in the microwave and cook for 8-9 minutes until the pudding has risen and has fully cooked through.

CONVERSION CHARTS

CONVERSION CHARTS

Volume

Imperial	Metric
1 tbsp	15ml
2 fl oz	55 ml
3 fl oz	75 ml
5 fl oz (¼ pint)	150 ml
10 fl oz (½ pint)	275 ml
1 pint	570 ml
1 ¼ pints	725 ml
1 ¾ pints	1 litre
2 pints	1.2 litres
2½ pints	1.5 litres
4 pints	2.25 litres

Cups	Imperial	Metric
1 cup flour	5oz	150g
1 cup caster or granulated sugar	8oz	225g
1 cup soft brown sugar	6oz	175g
1 cup soft butter/margarine	8oz	225g
1 cup sultanas/raisins	7oz	200g
1 cup currants	5oz	150g
1 cup ground almonds	4oz	110g
1 cup oats	4oz	110g
1 cup golden syrup/honey	12oz	350g
1 cup uncooked rice	7oz	200g
1 cup grated cheese	4oz	110g
1 stick butter	4oz	110g
¼ cup liquid (water, milk, oil etc)	4 tablespoons	60ml
½ cup liquid (water, milk, oil etc)	¼ pint	125ml
1 cup liquid (water, milk, oil etc)	½ pint	250ml

Oven temperatures

Gas Mark	Fahrenheit	Celsius
1/4	225	110
1/2	250	130
1	275	140
2	300	150
3	325	170
4	350	180
5	375	190
6	400	200
7	425	220
8	450	230
9	475	240

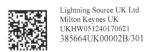